INTERMITTENT FASTING FOR WOMEN

Mastering fasting helps you lose weight and live
a healthy life

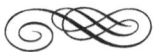

GILLIAN WILLET

Table of Contents

Introduction

Intermittent Fasting has become more popular than ever in the last few years!

There are lots of celebs, PTs and influencers who are singing its praises in terms of fat loss!

Many consider Intermittent Fasting to be a diet, but in reality it is not. It is simply a pattern of eating!

This pattern involves cycling between periods of eating and not eating. You only eat within certain time windows.

Intermittent fasting involves alternating periods of feast and famine in which you may eat as much as you like during the feasting, but drink only water during the fast. The aim is to achieve the benefits of calorie reduction and for some, use it as vehicle to lose weight.

Intermittent fasting can be done over a number of days, during alternating 24 hour periods or daily. The first option requires you abstain from some or all meals on one or more days of the week. Daily fasting utilizes 24 hour periods of eating and fasting that begin and end at the same time each day, for example fasting from Monday at 6 pm until Tuesday at 6 pm, eat as much as you like from Tuesday at 6 pm to Wednesday at 6 pm and repeat the process. During daily intermittent fasting there is a short period for eating, usually 4-6 hours within the 24 hour day during which you can eat as much as you like.

Some of the things that put people off are the fear they will be extremely hungry and not stick to the plan or they do not know how to fit it into their schedule. This is actually quite simple if you plan for it in advance. You get to eat your evening meal at pretty much the same time every day, but at an hour on either side depending if it is during an intermittent fasting phase or an eating phase. Again, with a little planning you can also accommodate socializing and eating out.

Intermittent fasting for women has some beneficial effects. What makes it especially important for women trying to lose weight is women have a much higher fat proportion in their bodies. When trying to lose weight, the body primarily burns through carbohydrate stores within the first 6 hours and then starts to burn fat. Women following a healthy diet and exercise plan may be struggling with stubborn fat, but fasting is a realistic solution to this.

Intermittent fasting can work but it's not for everyone, nor does it need to be. Intermittent fasting is just one approach, among many effective ones, for improving health, performance, and body composition.

A lot of people, especially women, now adopt intermittent fasting as an approach to lose body fat and it has now begun to gain more popularity.

An intermittent fasting weight loss program is radically different from most weight loss programs being promoted in the market. However, its ideas are scientifically sound when it comes to losing weight. You should give Intermittent Fasting a go if you are serious about weight loss.

Intermittent Fasting (If)

What is intermittent fasting (if)?

Intermittent Fasting (IF) refers to dietary eating patterns that involve not eating or severely restricting calories for a prolonged period of time. There are many different subgroups of intermittent fasting, each with individual variations in the duration of the fast; some for hours, others for day(s). This has become an extremely popular topic in the science community due to all of the potential benefits on fitness and health being discovered.

Fasting, or periods of voluntary abstinence from food has been practiced throughout the world for ages. Intermittent fasting with the goal of improving health is relatively new. Intermittent fasting involves restricting intake of food for a set period of time and does not include any changes to the actual foods you are eating. Currently, the most common IF protocols are a daily 16 hour fast and fasting for a whole day, one or two days per week.

Intermittent fasting could be considered as a natural eating pattern humans are built to implement and it can be traced all the way back to our Paleolithic hunter-gatherer ancestors. The current model of a planned program of intermittent fasting could potentially help improve many aspects of health from body composition to longevity and aging. Although IF goes against the norms of our culture and common daily routine, the science may be pointing to less meal frequency and more time fasting as the optimal alternative to the normal breakfast, lunch, and dinner model.

Intermittent fasting comes in various forms and each may have a specific set of unique benefits. Each form of intermittent fasting has variations in the fasting-to-eating ratio. The benefits and effectiveness of these different protocols may differ on an individual basis and so it is important to determine which one is best for you. Factors that may influence which one to choose include health goals, daily schedule/routine, and current health status.

Intermittent fasting is an effective tool for permanent fat loss, but it is important to keep in mind that everybody should adjust his fasting protocol to fit his individual body parameters to get rid of his excess fat as quickly as possible. Results of fasting are influenced by a person's volume of training and other physical activities, recovery capability and patterns, diet macronutrient ratios, exercise program type, eating habits and lifestyle, current body composition and daily lifestyle. That means you should start with a basic fasting program and monitor your results. Then you can tweak the program to fit your body needs to maximize getting rid of body fat.

The results of intermittent fasting are not limited to fat loss. Intermittent fasting can result also in a gain of lean muscle mass, health and performance improvements, better digestion of food, and improved immune function. an important benefit of fasting is improved insulin resistance, which is the foundation of the fat loss effect of fasting and metabolism improvement.

Intermittent Fasting Science

One of the most remarkable benefits of intermittent fasting is it has a positive effect on your mitochondrial networks, the fuel for your cells, by helping it remain fused. This undoubtedly improves energy, which can have positive effects on memory, longevity, and health challenges related to aging.

While intermittent fasting is trending, and many people are posting positive effects from their fasts, the research has mostly been conducted on mice.

The hope is that intermittent fasting isn't just a fad and that it has proven, lasting effects. Fasting research is on the rise. The hope is that more and more trials involving humans will be funded.

How Intermittent Fasting Works

Intermittent fasting is a controlled pattern of fasting made in an alternate way. Fasting? Meaning "not eat?" Yes, I really mean not to eat. Most of us when hungry chow down on any foods we can grab. This includes junk foods, processed foods and most of the time, fast foods. Anywhere we go, we see fast foods. Anywhere we go, we see street foods and so on. We eat three meals in a day and for most of us, three meals are not yet enough. We tend to feed ourselves more every time we feel any hunger or every time we feel the craving for food. We know very much that this is wrong, but we do not think of it and instead push ourselves to give in to that craving.

Regular meals are only breakfast, lunch and dinner. These are the only meals important to us. Every other meal is just additional and most of the time not needed, so it causes us to add to our weight and produce fat. When we do not work too much and we have a lot of physical activity then we might as well feed ourselves when hungry. But if we do not do much physical activity, then we should not give in to this temptous craving.

So what do we do?

This is where I can introduce intermittent fasting. This is where we eat our daily meals in a day and fast for the next twenty-four hours. We do not necessarily mean you cannot take in anything in your stomach. We just want you take in water or any healthy drink, including fruit juice. But we recommend that water is better.

Water does a lot of good things in our body. It cleans our body and helps flush out unhealthy food. There have been a lot of scientific studies and researches that proves intermittent fasting is very beneficial to our health. Remember, before now our ancestors did not have any fast foods, junk foods or street foods whenever they were hungry. What did they do? They drank water in order to quench their hunger. Most of the time, we feel hunger not because we really are hungry, but our body and mind just tells us to eat because it is used to doing so. We call this mental hunger. Sometimes, our minds just cheat us.

So this is the tip on intermittent fasting. Example, today you can eat as much food as you like. But be prepared that after dinner tonight you are just allowed to drink water afterwards for twenty-four hours. Drink water as much as you need to feed your hunger. This process will train your body and mind to not let you eat when you do not need to eat. This fasting will eventually lead your body to use the stored fat and energy that has not been used for a long period of time. So you will lose weight and stay healthier.

Intermittent fasting is not advisable for all people. This is only good for individuals without health problems. Whenever you wanted to try Intermittent fasting, you should consult first with your doctor before you push through.

Intermittent Fasting Myths

Unnatural and Unhealthy for the Body

One of the most prominent intermittent fasting myths is the idea that going without food is unnatural and potentially harmful for the body. This may be because our established dietary foundations have preached three square meals a day for so long. The traditional belief was that we need to constantly take in food to keep our metabolism burning hot.

What we know now is that this eating pattern will actually tend to promote weight gain, sugar cravings, and mood imbalances.

Times of fasting were relatively common for our ancestors. We have metabolic adaptation processes that occur to help us stay healthy during these times of scarcity. For example, the ability to produce energy from fats signifies that our bodies are well prepared to go long periods with no food.

In fact, intermittent fasting seems to have an overall healing effect on the body by stimulating repair and protection mechanisms.

Slows Down your Metabolism

As was mentioned already, most of us were raised on the idea that we need 3 square meals a day to keep our metabolism burning and blood sugar stable. If these meals are reliant on carbs and sugar as the primary source of calories, however, this eating pattern will tend to promote weight gain, insulin resistance, and an increased risk of heart disease.

Research shows intermittent fasting can actually have a metabolism boosting effect as it promotes a state of ketosis and increases growth hormone levels. What does slow down the metabolism is actually prolonged calorie restriction. This is why dieting in the traditional sense may not be a great idea.

This is one of the intermittent fasting myths that holds some weight, yet is easily resolved. All you need to do is ensure you are consuming enough calories to meet the metabolic demands of your body. There are several online tools that can help you estimate your metabolic rate.

Causes Nutrient Deficiencies

Fasting doesn't cause nutrient deficiencies, nutrient deficient diets do! If you are consuming a balanced whole foods diet within your eating window, it is unlikely you will suffer from any nutrient deficiencies.

If you are also following a ketogenic diet and/or consuming caffeine on a regular basis, you may need to hydrate more and consume more minerals by using a high-quality salt on your foods.

Other than that, there is very little reason for concern. Of all the intermittent fasting myths, this is one of the most unfounded. In fact, when you fast, your body develops a greater level of nutrient efficiency. When our blood sugar levels are going up and down, we drain much of our nutrient stores. When we fast, we use up significantly less nutrients and are able to retain them for future use.

If you are wondering how people develop micronutrient deficiencies then look at this chart and check out this article.

Causes Muscle Loss

One of the intermittent fasting myths originating from the fitness industry is intermittent fasting will lead to a loss of muscle mass. While it is true that the body will eventually revert to creating energy from muscle proteins during times of prolonged caloric restriction, this is unlikely to happen during a daily intermittent fast.

In fact, a recent study showed undergoing alternate-day fasting for a period of 8 weeks stimulated a fat loss on average of 12 lbs. while there was no significant loss in muscle mass. There is actually a protein sparing effect of fasting regularly, potentially from the stimulation of growth hormone.

If calories and protein intake are optimized within the eating window, you may actually be able to lose fat and gain muscle at the same time!

Causes Eating Disorders

Eating disorders are common in our society. If you feel like you struggle to incorporate healthy dietary choices on a daily basis, then intermittent fasting may not be for you just yet. I would recommend beginning with an anti-inflammatory nutrition plan as outlined here: 5 Benefits of a Healing Diet .

It is not likely intermittent fasting will cause an eating disorder. It is possible a dietary strategy aimed at promoting weight loss will attract those who already struggle with eating disorders, however.

To offer another perspective, constant obsession about food and impulsive eating habits are often largely caused by blood sugar imbalances. Following a ketogenic diet while employing intermittent fasting can go a long way in busting sugar cravings.

Some people will have the urge to binge eat following their fasting window, which could also be considered as an eating disorder. If your goal is weight loss and deriving the many health benefits from intermittent fasting, binge eating will inhibit these benefits.

Not Good for People with Diabetes

The idea that we need to eat constantly to maintain level blood sugar is an intermittent fasting myth that pervades the diabetic community as well. A recent study showed intermittent fasting improved weight loss, and fasting blood sugar, and helped to stabilize blood sugar after dinner in a group of type 2 diabetics.

In fact, prolonged fasting may even be able to restore insulin sensitivity in those suffering from type 2 diabetes. As an alternative or combination, following a ketogenic diet for a period of time can help to restore insulin sensitivity as well.

The better our insulin sensitivity, the less insulin our body will need to produce and the less inflammation our body will experience. This is very important for individuals with diabetes as it reduces their risk of heart disease and kidney failure.

For type I diabetics who cannot produce their own insulin, it is vital to closely monitor blood sugar to do this right. These individuals may still be able to fast for 12 and up to 16 hours daily depending upon how stable they are able to get their blood sugar levels.

Encourages Overeating

Blood sugar and leptin largely dictate our eating behaviors. If you have blood sugar instability, you will crave food when it comes crashing down. If you have become desensitized to leptin, you will have a hard time determining when you have had enough to eat.

Leptin is a signaling hormone in the body that largely controls your hunger levels. Poor sleep, stress, binge eating, and chronic calorie restriction can all contribute to leptin resistance, which will ultimately contribute to the tendency to overeat.

Intermittent fasting helps to improve blood sugar stability and leptin sensitivity which should improve impulse control over binge eating. If you are still struggling to overcome your cravings, you may find benefit in reading about a ketogenic diet and optimizing your dopamine levels:

You Shouldn't Exercise While Fasting

It is a common misconception that working out while fasting will lead to muscle wasting. What evidence shows is that, as long as adequate calories and protein are consumed on a daily basis, fasting workouts may actually boost muscle growth.

Additionally, there are a number of other benefits including improved fat burning, higher levels of growth hormone, the formation of new mitochondria, and an improved state of ketosis.

If you are going to perform high-intensity exercise while fasting on a regular basis, it will be important to ensure you are staying hydrated. If your goal is muscle gain, supplementing with essential amino acids can be very helpful as well.

You Will Feel Starved and Irritable

Many people fear this. They think when they fast, they will get super hungry and irritable. This is one of the fasting myths that may hold some weight, but only temporarily.

If you are accustomed to consuming three (or four, or five, etc.) periodically-spaced meals every day, you may feel a little irritable as you are adjusting to a new eating schedule. Start by performing simple fasts or just one 24 hour fast per week, on a Sunday for example. This is a great introduction to fasting most people find it easier than they expected. Start where you feel comfortable and work your way up. There is no rush to perform 16 hour fasts every day!

Once your body begins to adapt to going longer amounts of time without food, you may actually notice you feel best when you are fasting (no cravings or irritability at all). Many people take advantage of their heightened mental clarity during their fasting period every day to get some of their most challenging tasks done for the day!

It Will Cause Food Cravings

Food cravings are often a sign of low blood sugar or dopamine levels. While intermittent fasting may increase cravings for the first few days, in the long run it will help prevent them. Improved insulin sensitivity helps to stabilize blood sugar and ward off cravings as your body become metabolically flexible.

If you struggle with cravings throughout the morning, here's something else you can try: fat fasting.

Performing a fat fast during the morning can be excellent for mimicking a fast while staving off cravings. For coffee drinkers, I recommend Turmeric Fat Burning Coffee. For tea lovers, Keto

Matcha Green tea is excellent. If you are avoiding caffeine, you can try this Dandelion Coffee Alternative.

There are many intermittent fasting myths. Some have merit while others are simply wrong. Here I have laid out some of the most common myths and explained their shortcomings.

For most people, intermittent fasting has many benefits. This does not mean that everyone will thrive on the same style of fasting, however.

Benefits Of Intermittent Fasting

A large and growing body of medical research supports the use of intermittent fasting, showing it has a wide range of biological benefits. For example, intermittent fasting has been shown to:

1. Promote insulin sensitivity, which is crucial for your health, as insulin resistance or poor insulin sensitivity contributes to nearly all chronic diseases

2. Promote leptin sensitivity

3. Normalize ghrelin levels, also known as the "hunger hormone," resulting in lowered hunger

4. Improve blood sugar management by increasing insulin-mediated glucose uptake rates

5. Lower triglyceride levels

6. Increase human growth hormone production (HGH) — commonly referred to as "the fitness hormone." HGH plays an important role in maintaining health, fitness and longevity, including promotion of muscle growth, and boosting fat loss by revving up your metabolism. Research

shows fasting can raise HGH by as much as 1,300 percent in women and 2,000 percent in men.

The fact that it helps build muscle while simultaneously promoting fat loss explains why HGH helps you lose weight without sacrificing muscle mass, and why even athletes can benefit from intermittent fasting

7. Suppress inflammation and reduce oxidative damage

8. Upregulate autophagy and mitophagy, natural cleansing processes necessary for optimal cellular renewal and function

9. Boost fat burning and improve metabolic efficiency and body composition, including significant reductions in visceral fat and body weight in obese individuals

10. Prevent or reverse Type 2 diabetes, as well as slow its progression

11. Improve immune function

12. Lower blood pressure

13. Reduce your risk of heart disease — one study found those who fasted regularly had a 58 percent lower risk of coronary disease compared to those who never fasted

14. Reproduce some of the cardiovascular benefits associated with physical exercise

15. Boost mitochondrial energy efficiency and biosynthesis

16. Shift stem cells from a dormant state to a state of self-renewal

17. Reduce your risk of cancer

18. Increase longevity — there are a number of mechanisms contributing to this effect. Normalizing insulin sensitivity is a major one, but fasting also inhibits the mTOR pathway, which plays an important part in driving the aging process

19. Regenerate the pancreas and improve pancreatic function

20. Improve cognitive function, thanks to rising ketone levels

21. Protect against neurological diseases such as dementia, Alzheimer's disease and Parkinson's disease, thanks to the production of ketone bodies (byproducts of fatty acid breakdown, which are a healthy and preferred fuel for your brain) and brain-derived neurotrophic factor (BDNF, which activates brain stem cells to convert into new neurons, and triggers numerous other chemicals that promote neural health)

22. Eliminate sugar cravings as your body adapts to burning fat instead of sugar

Intermittent Fasting Considerations

While intermittent fasting is likely to be beneficial for most people, here are some points to consider:

- Intermittent fasting does not have to be a form of calorie restriction — it's a practice that should make you feel good. If your fasting strategy is making you feel weak and lethargic, you need to reevaluate your approach.

- Sugar cravings are temporary — your hunger and craving for sugar will slowly dissipate as your body starts burning fat as its primary fuel. Once your body has successfully shifted into fat burning mode, it will be easier for you to fast for as long as 18 hours and still feel satiated.

- It is not advisable to practice intermittent fasting if your daily diet is filled with processed foods — while intermittent fasting may sound like a panacea against ill health and excess weight, it alone may not provide you with all of these benefits. The quality of your diet plays an important role if you're looking for more than mere weight loss.

It's critical to avoid refined carbohydrates, sugar/fructose and grains. Focus your diet on vegetable carbohydrates, healthy protein in moderate amounts, and healthy fats such as butter, eggs, avocado, coconut oil, olive oil and raw nuts.

Considerations to Take Into Account before Embarking on Longer Fasts

This involves a base of intermittent fasting for 16 to 18 hours, and once or twice a week you have a 300- to 800-calorie meal loaded with detox supporting nutrients, followed by a 24-hour fast. So, in essence, you're then only eating one 300- to 800-calorie meal in 42 hours.

Using an infrared sauna and taking effective binders, like chlorella, modified citrus pectin, cilantro and even activated charcoal can help eliminate liberated toxins from your body and prevent their reabsorption. Gradually easing into longer fasts will also help minimize most side effects associated with fasting, as will transitioning over to a high-fat, low-carb diet, to help your body adjust to using fat as a primary fuel.

The so-called "keto flu" is often related to sodium deficiency, so it's recommended to use a high-quality unprocessed salt each day. This will also help reduce the likelihood of headaches and/or intractable muscle cramps at night. Another important mineral is magnesium. It's particularly important if you are diabetic, as magnesium deficiency is very common among Type 2 diabetics.

If you are taking medication, especially for your blood sugar, you have to make sure you talk to your doctor, because there's a risk your blood sugar may end up dipping too low. If you're taking insulin, and keep taking insulin while fasting, you could also get yourself into trouble.

If your doctor is adverse toward or unfamiliar with fasting, you'd be wise to find one that has some experience in this area so they can guide you on how to do this safely. There are also several absolute contraindications to water-only fasting. If any of the following apply to you, you should not do any extended types of fasting:

Underweight, defined as having a body mass index (BMI) of 18.5 or less.

Malnourished (in which case you need to eat healthier, more nutritious food).

Children should not fast for longer than 24 hours, as they need nutrients for continued growth. If your child needs to lose weight, a far safer and more appropriate approach is to cut out refined sugars and grains. Fasting is risky for children as it cuts out ALL nutrients, including those they need a steady supply of.

Pregnant and/or breastfeeding women. The mother needs a steady supply of nutrients in order to assure the baby's healthy growth and development, so fasting during pregnancy or while breastfeeding is simply too risky for the child.

Take Control of Your Health With Intermittent Fasting

Historically, generous amounts of food were not accessible throughout the entire year, let alone 24/7, and evidence shows you will radically increase your risk for chronic degenerative disease if you're keeping your body continuously fed.

"Adjustment of meal size and frequency has emerged as powerful tools to ameliorate and postpone the onset of disease and delay aging, whereas periods of fasting, with or without energy intake, can have profound health benefits.

The underlying physiological processes involve periodic shifts of metabolic fuel sources, promotion of repair mechanisms, and the optimization of energy utilization for cellular and organismal health.

Future research endeavors should be directed to the integration of a balanced nutritious diet with controlled meal size and patterns and periods of fasting to develop better strategies to prevent, postpone and treat the socio-economical burden of chronic diseases associated with aging.

In general, both prolonged reduction in daily caloric intake and periodic fasting cycles have the power to delay the onset of disease and increase longevity.

If you're new to the concept of intermittent fasting, consider starting by skipping breakfast; eat lunch and dinner within an eight-hour timeframe, and make sure you stop eating three hours before you go to sleep.

The latter is important, as it helps protect your mitochondrial function. Recent research shows men who eat supper at least two hours before bedtime have a 26 percent lower risk of prostate cancer, and women have a 16 percent lower risk of breast cancer than those who eat dinner closer to bedtime.

When you do eat, focus on healthy protein in moderate amounts, minimize net carbs like pasta and bread, exchanging them for healthy fats like butter, eggs, avocado, coconut oil, olive oil and raw nuts.

This will help shift you into fat burning mode. Remember, it may take a few weeks, but once you succeed, you may be easily able to fast for 18 hours and not feel hungry, making it that much easier to achieve your ideal weight. Virtually every aspect of your health will also begin to improve.

Types Of Intermittent Fasting

Intermittent fasting is a method of scheduled eating and fasting.

It's a way of scheduling your meals without changing what you eat.

Unlike other techniques like counting calories and limiting food intake, it doesn't make dieting a chore.

Research shows that counting calories causes stress, which can lead to an abandonment of the diet, feelings of deprivation, uncontrolled cravings, and weight regain.

On the other hand, intermittent fasting relies on time.

Rather than saying 'just eat less', a fixed rule of IF is not to eat after a certain time.

It is simple enough that anyone can do it and meaningful enough that it will serve its purpose.

In intermittent fasting, there is a fed state and a fasting state.

In the fed state, your body is digesting and absorbing food.

This starts when you begin eating and lasts for three to five hours as your body digests the food you ate.

This period is characterized by high insulin levels, which makes it very hard for your body to burn fat.

After this time, the body goes into the post-absorptive state.

It is when your body isn't processing your meal anymore.

This state lasts until 8 to 12 hours after your last meal.

The second state is now the fasting state when your insulin levels are low.

This makes it easier for your body to burn fat – even those that have been inaccessible during the fed state.

Simple And Painless Fast

The most cautious fast consists of no food restrictions, fasting one day per week, with only one meal on that day, and with a calorie intake at the 25 percent level (400 to 600 calories). On the other six days, eat normally.

5/2 Moderate Fast

The 5/2 fast consists of no food restrictions during two days per week, while reducing calorie intake to 25 percent, between 500 to 600 calories. On the other five days, you would eat normally.

Consistent Fasting

One of the most aggressive ways to intermittent fast is to adhere to your usual diet from 8 am to 3 pm, with fasting during the remaining hours of the day. On some days you might want a cheeseburger at 8 pm, but you can't have one.

Alternate-Day Fast

This intermittent fast might be one of the most difficult. Eating normally on one day and then fasting on the next day. To get the most benefit, you would continue this cycle somewhere between 8 and 16 weeks. Each fasting day can include 500 to 600 calories or no calories at all. In either case, be sure to drink plenty of water.

Alternate-day fasting can help you lose weight, and help lower your risk of heart disease and type 2 diabetes.

While restrictive, this diet tends to hold people's attention longer than most. The length of time that seems to produce the most benefits is 12 weeks, which is also the number of weeks that most human trials aim to achieve.

6/1 Fast

The 6/1 Fast is a simple fast where you eat nothing for one 24 hour period each week, starting with any meal (breakfast, lunch or dinner). During this time, doctors recommend that you drink plenty of water. Low-sugared coffee, tea, and other non-caloric and non-alcoholic beverages are permitted.

Keto Derivative

A form of The Keto Diet includes an aspect of intermittent fasting some people find helpful and effective. During every meal, eat your vegetables first and then eat your protein, with meals to be completed between 11 am to 6 pm, with intermittent fasting hours from 6 pm to 11 am. Refrain from heavy carbs like bread, pasta, and rice. Keep in mind that drastic reductions in carbs can make you feel a little foggy.

The Master Cleanse: Lemon Juice & Cayenne Pepper Fast

This popular fasting practice has been around since the 1940s, created by controversial figure, Stanley Burroughs. Stanley wrote The Master Cleanser in the 1940s, but the 1970s revision inspired a popular cleanse movement, which continues to this day. Fans of this cleanse include Beyoncé, Jared Leto, Denzel Washington, and Angelina Jolie.

The Master Cleanse consists of drinking only water mixed with a half-teaspoon of lemon juice and a hint of cayenne pepper 5 to 8 times per day, for 5 to 10 days.

While this fast is not recommended for everyone, and it's not a cure-all or intermittent fast, you might consider this idea when creating your own hybrid intermittent fast/diet.

One hybrid idea might be to drink this formula from 3 pm to 8 am and eat two calorie-restricted meals during the hours of 8 am to 3 pm.

The Warrior Diet

This intermittent fasting diet has some passionate followers. It involves fasting during the day and then eating a huge meal at night.

Popularized by fitness expert Ori Hofmekler, the dieter consumes small portions of raw fruits and raw vegetables during the day, then eats a high-calorie meal before 8 pm. In short, you fast all day (limited to fresh fruits and vegetables), and then you have a power-feast in the evening, finishing your banquet within a 4-hour eating window.

There are several challenges with this type of fasting. Depending on your body and metabolism, eating in the evening can extinguish the benefits of intermittent fasting. It might:

- Negatively impact your sleeping and dreaming patterns
- Alter hormone function
- Increase inflammation
- Impair blood sugar regulation
- Create weight gain
- Elevate triglycerides and cholesterol

Circadian Rhythm Or 16/8 Fasting

When it comes to losing weight, there are healthy and unhealthy paths. The Circadian Rhythm or 16/8 Fasting is when you eat solely during an 8-10 hour window each day. The rest of the time you refrain from meals and caloric beverages, but you can drink non-caloric, non-alcoholic drinks, including low-sugar coffee and tea.

Fitness expert and early promoter of intermittent fasting, Martin Berkhan called this diet, "The Leangains Protocol."

Intermittent Meal Plan Example

For this example, we'll focus on the 5/2 Intermittent Fast, which consists of two fasting days per week, each allowing 25 percent of your regular caloric intake (400 to 600 calories). When doing this fast, consider having an eating window from 8 am to 6 pm.

In addition to possibly losing addition weight, you'll have more food options if you avoid pieces of bread, rice, and pasta during your fast.

Here is an example of an under-600 calorie meal schedule:

Breakfast: 250 Calories

- 1/4 cup of oatmeal
- 8 oz Green smoothie with apples, spinach, and kale
- One hard-boiled egg or a one-egg Tex-Mex scramble with a pinch of tomatoes, onion, garlic, and salsa

Lunch/Dinner – 300 Calories

- One small baked potato with one tablespoon of sour cream
- 2 cups roasted vegetables with two tablespoons of hemp seeds
- 1/2 avocado on toast with one tablespoon of crushed peanuts or sesame seeds
- Chicken, Vegetable and Bean soup with 3 oz. of chicken, 1/4 cup of red beans, 1/2 cup of chopped veggies. You can swap

the chicken for 3 oz. of beef or buffalo, a moderate portion of tofu or 2 tablespoons of hemp seeds.

Between Meals – Under 60 calories (limited to one of these items, once per day)

- 2 cups of cooked microwave popcorn
- 1/2 cup cottage cheese
- Three whole grain pretzel sticks
- 14 almonds
- One apple (baked)
- 1/4 cup low-sugar ice cream
- 1/4-1/2 banana

Anytime

Water with 1/2 tsp of lemon juice and a tiny sprinkle of cayenne pepper. This drink is my favorite, especially during the fasting hours of 6 pm and 8 am or 6 pm and 11 am.

What To Eat During Intermittent Fasting

A popular misconception is you can allow yourself to eat anything while doing Intermittent Fasting, including fast food, sugary and highly processed dishes. If your goal is to lose weight, improve productivity and simply get healthier, it is important to stick to healthy meals.

This means eating whole foods and avoiding the usual suspects such as sugar, processed foods, empty carbs, etc.

The type of diet you choose is up to you, as long it is balanced and fits your lifestyle. For many, the Keto Diet has proven to be a great supplement to Intermittent Fasting as it may help you burn more fat.

1. Water

Even though you aren't eating, it's important to stay hydrated for so many reasons, like the health of basically every major organ in your body. The amount of water any one person should drink varies, but you want your urine to be a pale yellow color at all times. Dark yellow urine indicates dehydration, which can cause headaches, fatigue, and lightheadedness. Couple that with limited food, and it could be a recipe for disaster. If the thought of plain water doesn't excite you, add a squeeze of lemon juice, a few mint leaves, or cucumber slices to your water. It'll be our little secret.

2. Avocado

It may seem counterintuitive to eat the highest calorie fruit while trying to lose weight, but the monounsaturated fat in avocado is extremely satiating. A study even found that adding a half of an avocado to your lunch may keep you full for hours longer than if you didn't eat the green gem.

3. Fish

There's a reason the Dietary Guidelines suggests eating at least eight ounces of fish per week. Not only is it rich in healthy fats and protein, it also contains ample amounts of vitamin D. And if you're only eating a limited amount of food throughout the day, don't you want one that delivers more nutrient-bang for your buck? Not to mention that limiting your calorie intake may mess with your cognition, and fish is often considered a "brain food."

4. Cruciferous Veggies

Foods like broccoli, Brussels sprouts, and cauliflower are all full of the f-word—fiber. When you're eating erratically, it's crucial to eat fiber-rich foods that will keep you regular and prevent constipation. Fiber also has the ability to make you feel full, which is something you may want if you can't eat again for 16 hours.

5. Potatoes

Repeat after me: Not all white foods are bad. Case in point: Studies have found potatoes to be one of the most satiating foods around. Another study found that eating potatoes as part of a healthy diet could help with weight loss. Sorry, French fries and potato chips don't count.

5. Beans and Legumes

Your favorite addition to chili may be your best friend on the IF lifestyle. Food, specifically carbs, supplies energy for activity. While we're not telling you to carbo-load, it definitely wouldn't hurt to throw some low-calorie carbs, like beans and legumes, into your eating plan. Plus, foods like chickpeas, black beans, peas, and lentils have been shown to decrease body weight, even without calorie restriction.

6. Probiotics

You know what the little critters in your gut like the most? Consistency and diversity. That means they aren't happy when they're hungry. And when your gut isn't happy, you may experience some irritating side effects, like constipation. To counteract this unpleasantness, add probiotic-rich foods, like kefir, kombucha or kraut, to your diet. The Farmhouse Culture Gut Shots are perfect for any 500-calorie days, since each 1.5-ounce shot is brimming with live probiotics (10 billion CFUs) for just 10 calories.

7. Berries

Your favorite smoothie addition is ripe with vital nutrients. Strawberries are a great source of immune-boosting vitamin C, with more than 100 percent of the daily value in one cup. And that's not even the best part—a recent study found people who consumed a diet rich in flavonoids, like those in blueberries and strawberries, had smaller increases in BMI over a 14-year period than those who did not eat berries.

8. Eggs

One large egg has six grams of protein and cooks up in minutes. Getting as much protein as possible is important for keeping full and building muscle. One study found men who ate an egg breakfast instead of a bagel were less hungry and ate less throughout the day. In other words, when you're looking for something to do during your fasting period, why not hard-boil some eggs?

9. Nuts

They may be higher in calories than many other snacks, but nuts contain something that most junk food doesn't—good fat. Research suggests the polyunsaturated fat in walnuts can actually alter the physiological markers for hunger and satiety.

And if you're worried about calories, don't be! A 2012 study found that a one-ounce serving of almonds (about 23 nuts) has 20 percent fewer calories than listed on the label. Basically, the chewing process does not completely break down the almond cell walls, leaving a portion of the nut intact and unabsorbed during digestion.

10. Whole Grains

Being on a diet and eating carbs seem like they belong in two different buckets, but not always! Whole grains are rich in fiber and protein, so eating a little goes a long way in keeping you full. Plus, a new study suggests eating whole grains instead of refined grains may actually rev up your metabolism. So go ahead and eat your whole grains and venture out of your comfort zone to try farro, bulgur, spelt, kamut, amaranth, millet, sorghum, or freekeh.

What To Drink During Intermittent Fasting

To get all the health benefits of Intermittent Fasting such as fat loss, increased metabolic rate, lower blood sugar levels, boost in the immune system and others, you have to restrict from consuming any caloric food. But you can still consume non-caloric beverages because they do not break your fast and allow you to get all the benefits of fasting.

This is because non-caloric beverages do not cause the release of insulin and as a consequence, do not interfere with fat burning and/or autophagy (cellular cleanup).

1. Water

Water is always a great choice, all day long, every day. It can be still or sparkling, whatever you enjoy. You can also add a squeeze of lemon or lime to your water, or infuse a pitcher of water with cucumber or orange slices. But make sure you stay away from any artificially-sweetened water enhancers (like Crystal Light). The artificial sweetener will wreak havoc on your insulin levels, which defeats the entire purpose of fasting!

2. Coffee

Technically, black coffee is a calorie-free beverage, and many people drink it during fasting with no adverse effects. There are some people who experience a racing heart or upset stomach if they use coffee during a fast, so monitor your own experience. You can drink caffeinated or decaffeinated coffee, but any sweetener or milk is prohibited. Spices like cinnamon are totally fine!

Bonus: Black coffee might actually enhance some of the benefits of intermittent fasting. This study demonstrated that taking in caffeine can increase ketone production, which means you're more likely to slide into fat-burning mode even faster. Coffee has also been shown to improve your insulin sensitivity over the long term, which means more stable blood sugar.

3. Broths

A bone or vegetable broth is recommended for any time you decide to fast for 24 hours. Beware of canned broths or bouillon cubes, as these have tons of artificial flavors and preservatives that will counteract the effects of your fast. A good homemade broth, or one made by a trusted source, is the way to go.

4. Tea

Tea just might be the secret weapon that not only makes your fasting plan easier but also more successful. Read our primer on how to use tea to enhance your intermittent fasting plan.

All types of tea are great to drink during a fast, including green, black, oolong and herbal. But green tea, in particular, has been proven to help suppress appetite and enhance weight loss. And tea, in general, boosts the effectiveness of intermittent fasting by promoting gut health, probiotic balance, and cellular detoxification.

5. Apple Cider Vinegar

Drinking apple cider vinegar has numerous health benefits, and you can definitely continue drinking it while intermittent fasting. And since apple cider vinegar helps to regulate your blood sugar and improve your digestion, it actually enhances the effects of your intermittent fasting plan.

6. Drinks to Avoid

There are a few beverages that you might not realize are capable of breaking your fast. That just means that if you consume these, you will knock your body out of the fat-burning mode that intermittent fasting put you in: diet soda, coconut water, almond milk, and alcohol!

Even though diet soda technically doesn't have any calories, the artificial sweetener it contains will spike your insulin levels and wreak havoc with your blood sugar. Same goes for alcohol. And coconut water and almond milk both tend to be very high in sugar. Sugar equals carbs, so as soon as you consume these, you are no longer considered to be fasting.

Intermittent Fasting vs. Fad Liquid Diets

Intermittent fasting has been touted as a way to keep your mind sharp, regulate your weight and even extend your lifespan. The basic premise of this fast is to either eliminate solid food and drop your normal calorie count for two days per week, or eat within one eight-hour period per every 24 hours. For example, you would eat only between the hours of noon and 8 pm. This regimen is one that can be maintained indefinitely.

If you decide to choose the option of two consecutive days to fast, understand that it is not the fast itself that is beneficial — it is the change from regular eating to fasting and back again that seems to provide the benefits, which include increased mental focus and possible increased longevity. Simply limiting your caloric intake drastically will not work as a long-term weight-loss strategy, because your metabolism will adjust and start hoarding every calorie.

Fad liquid diets should be avoided, because they do not offer complete nutrition. The lemon juice, cayenne pepper and maple syrup craze may help you drop water weight, but after that your body will start to burn lean muscle mass. This diet is also very low in essential nutrients, and any weight you lose while on it will come right back once you resume your normal pattern of eating.

Stay away from commercially packaged shakes as well, because most contain huge amounts of sugar and can also be high in sodium. Your best bet for a liquid fast is to make smoothies at home, where you can control the calorie count and the quality of the ingredients.

Reasons To Practice Intermittent Fasting

Fasting is the practice of abstaining or reducing consumption of food, drink or both, for a specific period of time. Everyone fasts for at least some part of the day. Generally the eight or so hours one spends sleeping every night. Physiologically, fasting can refer to a person's metabolic status after not eating overnight or even the metabolic state after the complete digestion of a meal. Once you've gone 8 to 12 hours without eating, the body enters a state of "fasting." Intermittent fasting has many health benefits. Not least of which is weight loss, better skin, heart health and improved longevity. Jess Miller explains.

The practice of fasting can lead to a number of metabolic changes within the body. These changes typically begin approximately three to five hours after eating, when the body enters a "post-absorptive" state. Rather than the state of ongoing digestion. This is when eating frequent meals means the body is always involved in some sort of digestive activity.

Whether you practice more long-term fasting for health reasons or for spiritual reasons, most people will have to fast at some point for medical reasons. Patients undergoing surgery or other medical procedures requiring a general anaesthetic will usually fast prior to the treatment. In fact, individuals also practice fasting before undergoing a number of other medical tests. These include cholesterol testing, blood glucose measuring, or a lipid panel.

1. Weight Loss

Instead of running on fuel from the food you just ate, fasting allows your body to tap into its reserves. Fat which accumulates in the body is burned whenever the food supply grows scarce. This results in a slow, steady weight loss that can be a real benefit.

Since fasting is often incorporated as a lifestyle change instead of a temporary fix, this type of diet is much more sustainable than many other "crash diets." In fact, many studies support the practice as a valuable, reliable tool for weight loss and weight maintenance. Initially you'll see a marked weight loss as a result of losing water weight. However, according to the author of Eat Stop Eat, each day you fast will show a loss of 0.5 pounds of true body fat.

2. Improved Tolerance Of Glucose

For diabetics, fasting can be a fantastic way to normalize glucose and even improve glucose variability. Anyone looking for a natural way to increase insulin sensitivity should attempt an intermittent fast. The effects of fasting can make a difference in how your body processes glucose.

Generally, insulin resistance is the result of accumulation of glucose in tissues that aren't built for fat storage. As the body burns through stored fuel in the form of body fat, that excess accumulation becomes smaller and smaller. This allows the cells in your muscles and liver to grow increasingly responsive to insulin.

3. Boosts Metabolism

Part of the reason intermittent fasting helps you lose weight is the restriction of food, followed by regular eating, helps stimulate your metabolism. While long-term fasting can actually slow your metabolism, shorter fasts promoted by intermittent fasting have been proven to increase metabolism. In fact as much as up to 14 per cent, reported by one study.

This is also a more effective tool than long-term calorie restriction, which can often wreak havoc on the body's metabolism. Weight loss often goes hand in hand with muscle loss. And since muscle tissue is what burns through calories, having less muscle leads to a drop in your body's ability to metabolize food. Intermittent fasting keeps your metabolism running smoothly by helping you maintain your muscle tissue as much as possible.

4. Improves Longevity

Research has revealed intermittent fasting can "delay the development of disorders that lead to death. There's evidence people who fast regularly can enjoy a longer, healthier life than people who maintain a regular three meals a day lifestyle. Or those who follow a traditional restricted-calorie diet.

The mild stress that intermittent fasting puts on the body provides a constant threat. This increases the body's powerful cellular defenses against potential molecular damage. Intermittent fasting also stimulates the body to maintain and repair tissues. Its anti-aging benefits, keep every organ and cell functioning effectively and efficiently.

5. Understanding Hunger

It's important to learn how to accurately decipher the signals your body gives you. Intermittent fasting is a great way to understand the cycle of hunger. Before true hunger sets in and the body, if not fed, enters starvation mode, you'll feel pangs of "hunger" that can generally be attributed to psychological cravings. This emotional desire is confused with hunger all the time. Fasting will give you the opportunity to experience real "hunger pains" in the stomach, and even withdrawal and detox symptoms associated with our usual consumption of processed foods.

You'll also develop a deeper appreciation of food. If you've ever eaten after a period of "true hunger," you'll know what eating is supposed to feel like. Each bite tastes more delicious than the last, and you'll experience a sensation of deep contentment and pleasure. It's absolutely worth the hunger you endured to get here.

6. Establishes Routine

Unless you're following a random fasting type of diet, having strict eating times followed by periods of fasting can help your body develop a solid routine. You'll be able to recognize your own hunger cycles, sleep more soundly and start scheduling appointments during convenient hours. It can be difficult to establish this routine at first, especially if you have a family or an inflexible work schedule. However, once you've developed a consistent plan, you'll soon start to see all the ways a set routine can benefit your life and your health.

7. Stimulates Brain Function

Intermittent fasting may have "enormous implications for brain health." It showed fasting stimulates the brain in a number of different ways: promotes the growth of neurons, aids in recovery following a stroke or other brain injury, and enhances memory performance. Intermittent fasting may help decrease a practitioner's risk of developing neurodegenerative diseases like Parkinson's or Alzheimer's. There's also evidence to show that it may actually even improve both cognitive function and quality of life for people living with those conditions already.

8. Boosts The Immune System

Fasting has the power to "regenerate the entire immune system" by boosting the body's production of new white blood cells. This is how your body fights off infection. Fasting in cycles, enables your body to purge the damaged, old, or inefficient parts of the immune system, and replace them with newly generated immune system cells.

Studies showed that a 72 hour fast was even enough to help protect cancer patients from the harmful and toxic effects of chemotherapy treatments. These generally cause significant damage to the patient's immune system. Though researcher's need to conduct more clinical trials, many are confident that intermittent fasting could help immunocompromised individuals and the elderly.

9. Rejuvenates Skin

Acne sufferers know that one of the best ways to control bothersome skin conditions is through diet. Eating healthy, unprocessed foods and limiting the consumption of dairy products.

It's no surprise, then, that if you are a regular intermittent fasting practitioner, the impressive benefits will show all over your glowing, radiant face. Food sensitivities are often the root cause for many of these conditions which can lead to inflammatory conditions and acne. After a fast, you should introduce foods one at a time and note any changes to your skin, so that you can accurately pinpoint which foods you should avoid.

Intermittent fasting also has a positive effect on your hair and nails, helping them grow healthy and strong. Not only will you feel good after incorporating intermittent fasting into your lifestyle, you'll look great, too.

10. Improves Spiritual Well-Being

Almost every religion around the world practices fasting in one way or another. It's no surprise, then, that a lifestyle which includes intermittent fasting could lead to a deepened sense of spirituality. Regular practitioners have reported feeling at peace during their fasts. And studies have proven fasting can help regulate mood by reducing levels of anxiety and stress. In fact, fasting is a natural treatment many healthcare professionals recommend for a variety of emotional and sexual problems.

Whether or not you fast for religious reasons, intermittent fasting will help you feel more connected to nature and the world around you. And importantly you'll benefit from having a clearer mind and a more positive outlook.

Intermittent Fasting Mistakes That Could Make You Gain Weight

For most people, intermittent fasting works. When you fast, your body shifts its fuel source from glucose (either from incoming food or as a small amount of stored glycogen) to ketones or fat. In other words, your body literally utilizes body fat for fuel, making it ideal for fat burning without counting calories.

Equally important, intermittent fasting can create weight loss and fat loss while improving insulin sensitivity in overweight people. Fasting can also improve metabolic diseases such as type 2 diabetes while preserving muscle mass and function. It's even been shown to optimize your immune system, improve cognitive functioning and gut health, and help you sleep better.

But what if fasting doesn't work for you?

Maybe one of your favorite celebrities got big weight-loss results with intermittent fasting, or you read an article extolling fasting's benefits, so you decided to try it yourself. But you're sticking with the plan and not getting any of these benefits. You dutifully close the kitchen after dinner and skip breakfast the next morning, yet the scale refuses to budge, and you're always hungry at work.

So if you aren't getting the results you want, what's the point?

This can feel frustrating, but in many cases, something surprisingly simple could be holding you back. Consider whether any of these seven obstacles might be getting in your way of fasting success:

1. You don't journal.

Writing down what you eat (and don't eat) and tracking the hours you eat can pay dividends as you learn to maintain an intermittent fasting schedule. One study of almost 1,700 people found that writing down everything you eat could double weight loss. Tracking your food intake along with other measurements—your physical activity or mood levels, for instance—can also help you pinpoint potential obstacles to your success.

2. You're letting calories slip in during your fasting hours.

Fasting means consuming zero—or as close to zero—calories during your non-eating hours. You might have some not-so-obvious culprits slipping in that are breaking your fast. For some people, even a little bit of sweetener or cream in their coffee can knock them out of their fast and stall their results. Become aware of where these calories might be slipping in.

3. You're overeating.

Fasting typically helps you moderate your food intake without counting calories. One study looked at how people ate after a 36-hour fast. Researchers found while they ate slightly more calories at their next meal than non-fasters, they consumed almost 2,000 fewer calories over the two-day period. But for some people, breaking a fast can feel like an invitation to consume massive amounts of high-calorie food. Your body has to store those extra calories somewhere, and they usually form as fat—stalling your fasting results.

4. You're over-relying on coffee.

After doing an overnight fast, a big cup of organic dark roast can be the perfect start to your morning. Among its potential benefits, caffeine can dial down hunger while boosting energy levels. But using coffee as a crutch for poor sleep or managing your mood can mean you're drinking too much, which can contribute to weight gain over time in some people. Some research has shown that too much caffeine can increase blood glucose levels and prolong those increases, making you less insulin sensitive and more likely to store fat.

5. You're eating the wrong foods.

Fasting for 18 or even 24 hours doesn't give you permission to deep-dive into a deep-dish pizza or tip back a few glasses of wine during the hours you do eat. Those foods and drinks will spike and crash your insulin levels, sending you on a blood sugar roller coaster that leaves you hungry and moody during your fasting hours, potentially even stalling your results. When you eat matters, but so does what you eat. During your eating hours, ensure you're getting plenty of fiber, protein, and good fats from sources like vegetables, fruits, quality meats and fish, nuts and seeds, and olive oil.

6. You're moving too fast, too quickly.

Diving into a 24-hour fast immediately can become a full-blown disaster. Instead, start slowly with a smaller fasting window. Play with that window and gradually increase it (many people end up settling on an effective, yet sustainable 16:8 intermittent fasting schedule). Don't jump off the diving board before you're comfortable in the shallow end.

7. You're not maintaining stellar lifestyle habits.

What you eat and don't eat ultimately becomes an important piece of your healthcare puzzle. Just as important: Getting at least eight hours of stellar sleep nightly, managing stress levels, maintaining a healthy social and spiritual life, and consuming the right foods to support your fasting efforts and cultivate amazing health. When you maintain other good habits, you'll find fasting becomes easier and creates more lasting benefits.

Of course, no plan works for everyone, including fasting. If you're interested, give it a fair try: Commit to at least 30 days of fasting before you ultimately decide whether it works for you. (If you notice any adverse effects while fasting, please eat something and/or talk with your health care professional.)

How To Setup An Intermittent Fasting Diet

Establishing Eating / Fasting Times

The time of day in which you eat depends on if you are lifting weights that day, or not. On lifting days, your eating window is 9 hours and on the off or cardio days, its 6 hours. You will need to be able to weight train and do cardio at the same time of day, as this will throw off the schedule.

Eating schedule for weight training days

The fast is broken by a pre-workout shake, 15-30 minutes before you being your workout and lasts for 9 hours. For example, since I work out at 1 pm, my eating window begins at 12:30 pm and lasts until 9:30 pm. This can be inconvenient if you work out at say, 8 pm, so I feel weightlifting at lunchtime or in the morning works best.

Eating schedule for the off or cardio days

The fast is broken an hour after cardio is complete and lasts for 6 hours.

Summary

Monday: Fast ends at 12:30 pm and begins at 9:30 pm

Tuesday: Fast ends at 3:00 pm and begins at 9:00 pm

Wednesday: Fast ends at 12:30 pm and begins at 9:30 pm

Thursday: Fast ends at 3:00 pm and begins at 9:00 pm

Friday: Fast ends at 12:30 pm and begins at 9:30 pm

Saturday: Fast ends at 3:00 pm and begins at 9:00 pm

Sunday: Fast ends at 3:00 pm and begins at 9:00 pm

Determining Calories / Macronutrient Amounts:

Now that you have set up your eating / fasting schedule, it's time to figure out how many calories, as well as how much fat, carbohydrates and protein you will be eating. I realize that this might seem overwhelming at first, with all the math, but once you initially establish your requirements, it's really quite easy and routine.

Calories needed for Fat Loss

Caloric requirements depend on if it is a weight training day or an off/cardio only day.

To determine the number of calories needed for fat loss, you must first determine the calories needed for maintenance. The easiest way to get an estimate is to multiply your weight in pounds by 15. For example, if you weigh 200 lbs, the total calories needed for maintenance would be 3,000 calories per day.

Calorie requirements for weight training days:

To determine calories on weight training days, take the amount of maintenance calories and add 500 to it. So for our 200 lb person, they would be eating 3,500 calories on days that they lift.

Calorie requirements for the off or cardio days:

To determine the number of calories needed for the off or cardio days, simply divide your maintenance calories in half. So for the off or cardio days, our 200 lb person would be eating 1,500 calories per day.

Macronutrient Breakdown:

Now that your calorie requirements for fat loss have been determined, it's time to figure out how much of each macronutrient you will need. The amounts will vary depending on if you are weight training that day or not. The macronutrients we will be using, will be the big three:

* Fat

* Protein

* Carbohydrates

(Be sure to remember that fat has 9 calories per gram and protein and carbs each have 4 calories per gram.)

Macronutrient breakdown for weight training days:

Fat:

The maximum amount of fat eaten per day is 30 Grams. It doesn't matter where the fat comes from, as long as 10 of these grams are in the form of Omega-3 Fish Oil.

Protein:

To determine the minimum amount of protein per day, you multiply your weight by 1.25. Our 200 lb person will need a minimum of 250g of protein to preserve muscle. Sources don't really matter, just be sure to be mindful that you don't exceed the fat limit. Chicken, very lean red meat, fat free cheese and protein powder (whey or casein) are excellent choices.

Carbohydrates:

Carbohydrates make up the remaining calories in your diet. Once again, sources don't matter, just be sure not to exceed the 30g fat limit and be you want to keep sugar below 100 grams. So in our sample person, he is getting 270 calories from fat and 1,000 calories from protein. With the caloric goal on lifting days being 3,500, that leaves him with 2,230 calories left for carbs. Divide 2,230 by 4 and you come up with a maximum carbohydrate amount of ~558 grams.

Macronutrient breakdown for non-lifting or cardio days:

As mentioned earlier, calories needed for days that you don't weight train or do cardio are 1/2 of what your maintenance calories are. Here is the macronutrient breakdown:

Fat:

Again, the amount of fat is unchanged from training days. The maximum amount of fat eaten per day is 30 Grams. It doesn't matter where the fat comes from, as long as 10 of these grams are in the form of Omega-3 Fish Oil.

Carbohydrates:

On rest days or cardio only days, carbohydrate sources should only come from fibrous green vegetables and the trace amounts found in your protein sources, such as whey and cheese. The maximum amount per day should not exceed 20 grams.

Protein:

The minimum amount of protein is your weight in pounds x 1.25. For our sample person requiring 1,500 calories per day, he would be getting 270 calories from fat, 80 calories from carbohydrates and the remaining 1,150 calories from protein. That would equal to ~287.5 grams.

Diet for Weight Training Days

Weight training will be a 3 day a week, full body routine. The days are up to you, as long as there is a day off between workouts. Keep reading for my workout recommendation.

Pre-Workout

On training days, the fast is broken with a whey protein/carb shake, 15-30 minutes before your workout begins.

I suggest a mix of simple carbs and whey protein.

Protein =.25g/lb x weight Carbs =.25g/lb x weight

Gatorade powder (not the pre-made liquid form) or a maltodextrine/dextrose blend is my pre-workout carb of choice. Keep fat to a minimum here.

Post-Workout

Within 30 minutes of your workout, you have another shake, but this time, use a whey + casein/dextrose mix.

Protein =.25g/lb x weight Carbs =.50g/lb x weight

The Rest of the day

Your first solid food meal of the day is 1 hour after your PWO shake. This will be the biggest meal of the day. Remaining meal times are up to you, but I recommend tapering your calories down until your last meal. Remember, with Intermittent Fasting, you don't need to eat every 2-3 hours. Just make sure that you meet your caloric/macronutrient goals. I do however, recommend a casein shake right before the eating period is over. Since it's a slow digesting protein, it will help keep you full longer.

Diet for Off or Cardio Days

Since calories are greatly reduced on off or cardio days, the eating window is shorter. It works best to have 2-3 good size meals, rather than the 6-7 you read about in muscle mags.

On cardio days, the fast is broken with a 50g protein shake, 1 hour after cardio is complete. Two hours after the shake, have your first "real" meal and continue until the 6 hours are up. As I mentioned earlier, carbs are limited to 20 per day and should consist of fibrous green vegetables and the trace amounts in food.

Intermittent Fasting Diet Weight Training Routine

Weight training is a full body 3 day routine. Again, exact days don't really matter, but make sure you have a day off in between workouts. You will be working the large muscles only (legs, back, chest) on days 1 and 2 and will add in the smaller muscles arms/calves) on day 3. You will do 4 sets of 6-8 reps for each large muscle and 2-3 sets of 8-12 for the smaller ones.

Here is a sample workout routine:

Day 1: Push

Flat Bench Press / Shoulder Press / Leg Press / Weighted Crunches

Day 2: Pull

Rows / Chin-ups / Hamstring Curl

Day 3: Push/Pull

Incline Bench Press / Rows / Squats / Calf Raises / Lateral Raise / Barbell Curl / Triceps Pushdown / Lateral Raise / Back Extensions / Weighted Crunches

For maximum fat loss, cardio should be down 2-3 times per week. Start with a 5 minute warm-up and then begin 10 minutes of High Intensity Interval Training, or HIIT. This works best on an elliptical or a spin bike, instead of a treadmill. You will do this in 1 minute intervals. Max intensity for 1 minute, followed by a moderate pace for 1 minute. Repeat until 10 minutes are up. After the HIIT session is over, drink some water and rest for 5 minutes. After your rest, do 30 minutes of Low to Moderate Intensity, Steady State Cardio. A treadmill works great for this. Don't forget to wait an hour and have your 50g of protein.

The Beginner's Guide To Intermittent Fasting

Intermittent fasting is not a diet, it's a pattern of eating. It's a way of scheduling your meals so you get the most out of them. Intermittent fasting doesn't change what you eat, it changes when you eat.

Why is it worthwhile to change when you're eating?

Well, most notably, it's a great way to get lean without going on a crazy diet or cutting your calories down to nothing. In fact, most of the time you'll try to keep your calories the same when you start intermittent fasting. (Most people eat bigger meals during a shorter time frame.) Additionally, intermittent fasting is a good way to keep muscle mass on while getting lean.

With all that said, the main reason people try intermittent fasting is to lose fat. We'll talk about how intermittent fasting leads to fat loss in a moment.

Perhaps most importantly, intermittent fasting is one of the simplest strategies we have for taking bad weight off while keeping good weight on because it requires very little behavior change. This is a very good thing because it means intermittent fasting falls into the category of "simple enough so you'll actually do it, but meaningful enough it will actually make a difference."

How Does Intermittent Fasting Work?

To understand how intermittent fasting leads to fat loss we first need to understand the difference between the fed state and the fasting state.

Your body is in the fed state when it is digesting and absorbing food. Typically, the fed state starts when you begin eating and lasts for three to five hours as your body digests and absorbs the food you just ate. When you are in the fed state, it's very hard for your body to burn fat because your insulin levels are high.

After that time span, your body goes into what is known as the post–absorptive state, which is just a fancy way of saying that your body isn't processing a meal. The post–absorptive state lasts until 8 to 12 hours after your last meal, which is when you enter the fasted state. It is much easier for your body to burn fat in the fasteing state because your insulin levels are low.

When you're in the fasting state your body can burn fat that has been inaccessible during the fed state.

Because we don't enter the fasting state until 12 hours after our last meal, it's rare that our bodies are in this fat burning state. This is one of the reasons why many people who start intermittent fasting will lose fat without changing what they eat, how much they eat, or how often they exercise. Fasting puts your body in a fat burning state which you rarely make it to during a normal eating schedule.

The Benefits Of Intermittent Fasting

1. Intermittent fasting helps you live longer.

Scientists have long known that restricting calories is a way of lengthening life. From a logical standpoint, this makes sense. When you're starving, your body finds ways to extend your life.

There's just one problem: who wants to starve themselves in the name of living longer?

The good news is intermittent fasting activates many of the same mechanisms for extending life as calorie restriction. In other words, you get the benefits of a longer life without the hassle of starving.

Way back in 1945 it was discovered intermittent fasting extended life in mice. More recently, this study found alternate day intermittent fasting led to a longer lifespan.

2. Intermittent fasting may reduce the risk of cancer.

This one is up for debate because there hasn't been a lot of research and experimentation done on the relationship between cancer and fasting. Early reports, however, look positive.

This study of 10 cancer patients suggests that the side effects of chemotherapy may be diminished by fasting before treatment. This finding is also supported by another study which used alternate day fasting with cancer patients and concluded fasting before chemotherapy resulted in better cure rates and fewer deaths.

Finally, this comprehensive analysis of many studies on fasting and disease has concluded fasting appears to not only reduce the risk of cancer, but also cardiovascular disease.

3. Intermittent fasting is much easier than dieting.

The reason most diets fail isn't because we switch to the wrong foods, it's because we don't actually follow the diet over the long-term. It's not a nutrition problem, it's a behavior change problem.

This is where intermittent fasting shines because it's remarkably easy to implement once you get over the idea you need to eat all the time. For example, this study found intermittent fasting was an effective strategy for weight loss in obese adults and concluded "subjects quickly adapt" to an intermittent fasting routine.

"Diets are easy in the contemplation, difficult in the execution. Intermittent fasting is just the opposite — it's difficult in the contemplation, but easy in the execution.

Most of us have contemplated going on a diet. When we find a diet that appeals to us, it seems as if it will be a breeze to do. But when we get into the nitty gritty of it, it becomes tough.

Intermittent fasting is hard in the contemplation, of that there is no doubt. "You go without food for 24 hours?" people would ask, incredulously when we explained what we were doing. "I could never do that." But once started, it's a snap. No worries about what and where to eat for one or two out of the three meals per day. It's a great liberation. Your food expenditures plummet. And you're not particularly hungry. ... Although it's tough to overcome the idea of going without food, once you begin the regimen, nothing could be easier."

In my opinion, the ease of intermittent fasting is best reason to give it a try. It provides a wide range of health benefits without requiring a massive lifestyle change.

Examples of Different Intermittent Fasting Schedules

If you're considering giving fasting a shot, there are a few different options for working it into your lifestyle.

Daily Intermittent Fasting

This model of daily intermittent fasting was popularized by Martin Berkhan of Leangains.com, which is where the name originated.

It doesn't matter when you start your 8–hour eating period. You can start at 8 am and stop at 4 pm. Or you start at 2 pm and stop at 10 pm. Do whatever works for you.

Lean gains of daily intermittent fasting

Because daily intermittent fasting is done every day it becomes very easy to get into the habit of eating on this schedule. Right now, you're probably eating around the same time every day without thinking about it. Well, with daily intermittent fasting it's the same thing, you just learn to not eat at certain times, which is remarkably easy.

One potential disadvantage of this schedule is because you typically cut out a meal or two out of your day, it becomes more difficult to get the same number of calories in during the week. Put simply, it's tough to teach yourself to eat bigger meals on a consistent basis. The result is many people who try this style of intermittent fasting end up losing weight. That can be a good thing or a bad thing, depending on your goals.

Weekly Intermittent Fasting

One of the best ways to get started with intermittent fasting is to do it once per week or once per month. The occasional fast has been shown to lead to many of the benefits of fasting we've already talked about, so even if you don't use it to cut down on calories consistently there are still many other health benefits of fasting.

For example, lunch on Monday is your last meal of the day. You then fast until lunch on Tuesday. This schedule has the advantage of allowing you to eat every day of the week while still reaping the benefits of fasting for 24 hours. It's also less likely you'll lose weight because you are only cutting out two meals per week. So, if you're looking to bulk up or keep weight on, then this is a great option.

There are a wide range of variations and options for making it work into your schedule. For example, a long day of travel or the day after a big holiday feast are often great times to throw in a 24–hour fast.

Perhaps the biggest benefit of doing a 24–hour fast is getting over the mental barrier of fasting. If you've never fasted before, successfully completing your first one helps you realize you won't die if you don't eat for a day.

Alternate Day Intermittent Fasting

Alternate day intermittent fasting incorporates longer fasting periods on alternating days throughout the week.

For example, you would eat dinner on Monday night and then not eat again until Tuesday evening. On Wednesday, however, you would eat all day and then start the 24–hour fasting cycle again after dinner on Wednesday evening. This allows you to get long fast periods on a consistent basis while also eating at least one meal every day of the week.

The benefit of alternate day intermittent fasting is that it gives you longer time in the fasted state than the Leangains style of fasting. Hypothetically, this would increase the benefits of fasting.

Teaching yourself to consistently eat more is one of the harder parts of intermittent fasting. You might be able to feast for a meal, but learning to do so every day of the week takes a little bit of planning, a lot of cooking, and consistent eating. The end result is most people who try intermittent fasting end up losing some weight because the size of their meals remains similar even though a few meals are being cut out each week.

If you're looking to lose weight, this isn't a problem. And even if you're happy with your weight, this won't prove to be too much of an issue if you follow the daily fasting or weekly fasting schedules. However, if you're fasting for 24 hours per day on multiple days per week, then it's going to be very difficult to eat enough of your feast days to make up for that.

Frequently Asked Questions

I could never skip breakfast. How do you do it?

If you eat a big dinner the night before, you'll be surprised by how much energy you have in the morning. Most of the worries or concerns people have about intermittent fasting are due to the fact they have had it pounded into them by companies they need to eat breakfast or they need to eat every three hours and so on. The science doesn't support it and neither do my personal experiences.

I thought you were supposed to eat every 3 hours?

You may have heard people say you should have six meals per day or eat every 3 hours or something like that.

Here's why this was a popular idea for a brief period of time:

Your body burns calories when it's processing food. So the thought behind the more meals strategy was if you ate more frequently, you would also burn more calories throughout the day. Thus, eating more meals should help you lose weight.

Here's the problem:

The amount of calories you burn is proportional to the size of the meal your body is processing. So, digesting six smaller meals that add up to 2,000 calories burns the same amount of energy as processing two large meals of 1,000 calories each.

It doesn't matter if you get your calories in 10 meals or in 1 meal, you'll end up in the same place.

This is crazy. If I didn't eat for 24 hours, I'd die.

Mental barrier is the biggest thing that prevents people from fasting because it's really not that hard to do in practice.

Here are a few reasons why intermittent fasting isn't as crazy as you think it is.

First, fasting has been practiced by various religious groups for centuries. Medical practitioners have also noted the health benefits of fasting for thousands of years. In other words, fasting isn't some new fad or crazy marketing ploy. It's been around for a long time and it actually works.

Second, fasting seems foreign to many of us simply because nobody talks about it that much. The reason for this is nobody stands to make much money by telling you to not eat their products, not take their supplements, or not buy their goods. In other words, fasting isn't a very marketable topic and so you're not exposed to advertising and marketing on it very often. The result is it seems somewhat extreme or strange, even though it's really not.

Third, you've probably already fasted many times, even though you don't know it. Have you ever slept in late on the weekends and then had a late brunch? Some people do this every weekend. In situations like these, we often eat dinner the night before and then don't eat until 11 am or noon or even later. There's your 16–hour fast and you didn't even think about it.

The 1-Week Intermittent Fasting Meal Plan

Intermittent fasting is something so many people have heard about, but perhaps may not totally understand what it is or how to implement it. Essentially, intermittent fasting is a conscious decision to only eat during certain periods of the day. It's not technically a diet because it doesn't limit what you can eat. However, you do have to be mindful of the types of foods you choose. These meals will have to get you through the rest of the day. Whether you've been intermittent fasting for years or just interested in what it looks like, check out this intermittent fasting meal plan.

Before we begin the intermittent fasting meal plan, it's important to understand why intermittent fasting is different than just regular fasting. While there are a variety of ways people approach this, usually people follow a 16/8 strategy which involves eating 8 hours a day and fasting for the other 16 hours. However, there are numerous strategies people may follow. The point is to have a period of time in which a person is not consuming calories and then when they do eat, they avoid processed foods and focus on whole food recipes.

Many people choose to skip breakfast or dinner, but the method doesn't necessarily require you skip meals. You should also recognize the specific caloric intake may vary based on your body's needs to lose weight. Generally, you should focus on eating meals including fish, lean meats, whole grains, and plenty of veggies. The idea here is you'll eat a couple of larger meals, but your caloric intake will actually be lower because you will only be consuming foods within a certain timeframe.

Day 1

> Breakfast: Spinach Parmesan Baked Eggs
>
> Lunch: Oven-Crisp Fish Tacos
>
> Dinner: Turkey Burrito Skillet
>
> Snack: Dark Chocolate (suggested two squares)

Day 2

> Breakfast: Hummus Breakfast Bowl
>
> Lunch: Baked Lemon Salmon and Asparagus Foil Pack

Dinner: Chicken and Broccoli Stir Fry

Snack: Boiled egg

Day 3

Breakfast: 4-Ingredient Protein Pancakes

Lunch: Wild Cod with Moroccan Couscous

Dinner: Honey Garlic Shrimp Stir Fry

Snack: Almonds (suggested 12-14)

Day 4

Breakfast: Ham and Egg Breakfast Cups

Lunch: Sweet Potato and Turkey Skillet

Dinner: Savory Lemon White Fish Fillets

Snack: Two stalks of celery with peanut butter

Day 5

Breakfast: No-Bake Oatmeal Raisin Energy Bites

Lunch: Cucumber Quinoa Salad with Ground Turkey, Olives, Feta

Dinner: Skinny Salmon, Kale, and Cashew Bowl

Snack: 1 cup fresh strawberries

Day 6

Breakfast: Creamy Green Smoothie with a Hint of Mint

Lunch: Baked Chicken and Vegetable Spring Rolls

Dinner: Skinny Turkey Meatloaf

Snack: Avocado and tomatoes

Day 7

Breakfast: Sweet Potato Breakfast Hash

Lunch: Spicy Black Bean and Shrimp Salad

Dinner: Turkey Sausage with Pepper and Onions

Snack: Two cups of chopped celery and carrots

Keep in mind, the specifics for your diet will vary based on how many calories you should be taking in for weight loss. You'll need to calculate your required calorie intake in order for a meal plan to be most effective.

Experiments With Intermittent Fasting

1. First, decide if it's right for you.

Although there are some neat benefits, IF is not for everyone. Your exercise and nutritional experience, and your lifestyle, should determine whether you try IF. If you're new to exercise and nutrition, I strongly recommend you learn the essentials first.

2. Start slowly. Start simply. Start small. Start gradually.

If you decide you'd like to try IF, there's no rush. Pick one small thing to try, even if that's just adjusting regular mealtimes by an hour. Try it. See how it goes.

3. Focus on what IF approaches have in common, rather than getting bogged down in the details.

Sometimes you eat. Sometimes you don't. That pretty much sums it up.

4. Stay flexible.

5. Know thyself. Observe your own experiences carefully.

Be a scientist. Get started, gather data, gain insight, and draw conclusions that you use to guide future action. Do what's right for you.

6. Give it time.

There is no rush. Especially since it usually takes a few weeks just to adapt to your new program.

7. Expect ups and downs.

They happen, it's part of life, and it's part of the process. By staying open-minded and not panicking during the "downs" you'll figure out how to have more "ups."

8. Think about what you truly want from IF. Focus on the quality of the process, not the outcome.

IF is a great way to:

Go deeper into the psychological and physical experience of true hunger;

learn the difference between "head hunger" and "body hunger;"

learn not to fear hunger;

improve insulin sensitivity and re-calibrate your body's use of stored fuel;

respect the process and privilege of eating;

learn more about your own body;

lose fat, if you are careful about it; and,

take a break from the work of food prep and the obligation to eat.

IF is not healthy if:

You're using the pretext of "health" as a way to have an eating disorder and/or rigidly control your food intake (which is really the same thing);

you fast too often, too long;

you're also over-exercising or not getting enough sleep (i.e., under too much additional physiological stress);

you're using a lot of supplements, legal or otherwise, to kill your appetite so you can make it through your fasts;

you're food-obsessed and/or binge during your non-fasting periods; and, you use IF as a way to "compensate" for poor food choices or over-eating.

9. What you DO eat is as important as what you DON'T.

Get the nutritional basics down first. Eat good quality food, in the right amounts, at the right times. For most people, this is enough to get into great shape. No IF required.

For more on this, see our 5-Day Fat Loss course, in the resources section.

10. Respect your body cues.

Pay attention to what your body tells you.

This includes:

drastic changes in appetite, hunger, and satiety – including food cravings;

sleep quality;

energy levels and athletic performance;

mood and mental/emotional health;

immunity;

blood profile;

hormonal health; and,

how you look.

11. Exercise, but don't overdo it.

We strongly recommend you combine exercise with IF to get the most out of it. Just don't overdo it.

12. Consider what else is going on in your life.

Think about:

how much exercise/training you do, and how intensely;

how well you rest and recover;

how well IF is fitting into your regular routine and normal social activities; and,

what other demands and stress life offers you.

Remember: IF is one of many nutrition styles that work. But it only "works" when it's intermittent, flexible, and part of your normal routine – not an obligation, and not a chronic source of physical and psychological stress.

Dos And Don'ts Of Intermittent Fasting

Dos of Intermittent Fasting

Intermittent Fasting requires these steps to be followed to gain the maximum benefit out of it.

Consult with a Doctor

Regularly consulting with your doctor is an essential part of intermittent Fasting. Always try to follow the suggestions of your physician and avoid trying it with your own ideas, which may lead to harmful side-effects.

Plan your Fasting Schedule

Those who fail to plan, plan to fail. Out of your daily routine, pick an appropriate period of time to do an intermittent fast. The best way to design a plan for intermittent fast is to consult a doctor.

Ask the doctor to analyze your current body weight and calorie intake to suggest the right fasting plan for you.

During eating hours, try to follow the diet plan suggested by your doctor and avoid taking in calorie-enriched food.

Stay Hydrated

You don't want to turn into a cactus!

While you are restricting calorie intake, make sure you continue to drink water. Drinking water will give your body a cleanse and purify the blood vessels.

If, for some reason, you are not able to drink water in a large enough quantity, try to take fruits and their juices that contain a large amount of water such as orange and watermelon. Other than water, tea, black coffee, and natural juices are also good supplements to keep you hydrated.

Monitor your Body's Reactions

Keep a close eye on your body conditions. Try to keep the weekly track of your body weight; it will help you to make a comparison and make decisions accordingly. Most people feel uncomfortable and fatigued when trying intermediate fasting for the first time.

Always make sure that you don't over-do it to lose weight. You probably know someone who started out doing intermediate fasting and then it started turning into anorexia.

Do intermittent fasting to the extent at which you would be able to complete your everyday work with ease.

Take Vitamins

Intermittent fasting can be the cause of reduced vitamins in your body. To avoid this condition, take supplementary vitamins according to the suggestion of the doctor.

Along with supplements, eat fruits that have large amounts of vitamins and minerals. Avoid artificially-sweetened products.

Relax and Enjoy the Fun

It is tough for a person to spend time their time dreaming about all of the donuts or hamburgers they could be eating during an Intermittent Fast. It can lead to irritation, stress, and sometimes depression.

Avoid this by getting involved in fun activities and having discussions with your friends. Try not to be alone and bored during your fast. It should be a happy time.

Don'ts of Intermittent Fasting

To maximize the effect of Intermittent Fast, stay away from the things discussed below.

Don't overeat before Fasting

According to the experts, it is strongly discouraged to eat a heavy meal before fasting.

It may be injurious to your health, especially to your stomach, because of the slow burning nutrition in heavy or oily foods.

Always try to take in low-calories and average-protein meal before fasting. At night, and have some natural sugar fruits like apple, mango, watermelon, etc.

Don't Push too hard

If you feel ill or severely fatigued while fasting, give your body the priority in front of your Intermittent Fast.

The experts warn against fasting with health conditions like diabetes, cancer, and pregnancy. These conditions require precise steps to be followed. Consultation with a doctor is crucial for individuals with these health situations.

Don't be Stressed Out

Be calm and cool. Stress can raise the level of cholesterol in your body. Fasting is not ideal if it is causing abnormal stress levels in the body. Yoga and deep breathing are good practices to attain relief from stress.

Don't Exercise Heavily

Exercises like yoga and jogging are always encouraged to practice while you are fasting.

Remember that your energy level is lower while in the fasting state. It, therefore, goes without saying that you don't want to lift excessive weights or run a marathon in this state. Be practical with lighter exercise.

Who Should And Who Should Not Practice Intermittent Fasting

Intermittent fasting (IF) may sound technical. But all it really means is going for extended periods without eating.

Why would anybody want to do that? Well, a growing number of fitness experts claim that the practice can help people lose fat and improve their health.

But intermittent fasting is hardly the exclusive preserve of nutrition nerds. In fact, we all do some form of it every single day. Except we don't call it that. We call it sleeping.

That's right. The time from your last meal at night until your first meal the next day could be described as a "fasting" interval.

(And the time from your first meal of the day until your last meal can be called a "feeding" interval.)

It's as simple as that. So try not to get too entranced by the terminology.

In the end, people who decide to practice intermittent fasting simply extend the length of time when they are not eating.

Of course, everyone's jockeying to "get it right." Which means many different protocols have emerged -- Eat Stop Eat, Leangains, the Warrior Diet, the 5:2 diet, and more -- but in one way or another, all of these plans shrink the "eating" window and expand the "not eating" window.

What's the point of fasting?

Although the name may be a recent invention, intermittent fasting is nothing new. In fact, humans have always fasted, whether just overnight, during more extended periods of food scarcity, or for religious reasons.

Data suggest that IF, when done properly, might help extend life, regulate blood glucose, control blood lipids, reduce the risk of coronary disease, manage body weight, help us gain (or maintain) lean mass, reduce the risk of cancer, and more.

Now, these studies are still in their early stages, so there's plenty of room for skepticism. Still, some of the findings look promising.

That's why many people in the fitness world have decided to put IF to the test. In the absence of hard data, they're opting for personal experimentation.

But intermittent fasting is not for everyone

While intermittent fasting worked for some, it is not a good fit for everybody.

First of all, intermittent fasting is not just another way of saying "free ride." Randomly skipping meals while continuing to eat a diet high in processed foods won't help you lose fat or improve your health.

So while there's no one "right" way to practice fasting, any decent protocol will involve a certain amount of attention to nutritional specifics. You have to be prepared to do that work.

Some will find IF too inconvenient or troublesome to practice. And for others, its risks far outweigh any potential benefits. In fact, for some people IF could be downright dangerous.

Before you skip your next meal, you probably want to know whether you fall into that category.

Here's the lowdown, based on numerous case studies and a small amount of published research.

You're most likely to be successful with intermittent fasting if:

- You have a history of monitoring calorie and food intake (e.g., you've "dieted" before)
- you're already an experienced exerciser
- You're single or you don't have children
- Your partner (if you have one) is extremely supportive
- Your job allows you to have periods of low performance while you adapt to a new plan
- You're male

The first five factors will allow you to build the protocols into your lifestyle more easily, while the final condition (being male) seems to affect results.

Meanwhile, if you meet the following criteria, you may want to proceed with caution:

- You're married or have children
- You have performance oriented or client-facing jobs
- You compete in sport/athletics
- You're female

Again, the first three conditions make it much harder to follow IF protocols and may make it impractical for you. What's more, trying to fast may conflict with performance goals for your sport.

As for the last condition, some experimenters suggest that for women, fasting causes sleeplessness, anxiety, irregular periods, and other indications of hormone dysregulation.

In particular, women seem to fare worse on the stricter forms of intermittent fasting than men do. So if you're female and you want to try fasting, I recommend beginning with a very relaxed approach.

Finally, there are some people who really shouldn't bother with intermittent fasting at all. Don't try it if:

- You're pregnant
- You have a history of disordered eating
- You are chronically stressed
- You don't sleep well
- You're new to diet and exercise

If you're new to diet and exercise, intermittent fasting might look like a magic bullet for weight loss. But you'd be a lot smarter to address any nutritional deficiencies before you start experimenting with fasts. Ensure you're starting from a solid nutritional platform first.

Pregnant women have extra energy needs, so if you're starting a family, this is not the time to fast.

Ditto if you are under chronic stress and/ or not sleeping. Your body needs nurturing, not additional stress.

And if you've struggled with disordered eating in the past, you probably recognize a fasting protocol could lead you down a path that might create further problems for you. Why mess with your health? You can achieve similar benefits in other ways.

Cook and eat whole foods. Exercise regularly. Stay consistent. And if you'd like some help to do all of that, find a mentor or coach.

Heck, that last part is relevant even if you decide to try intermittent fasting.

While self-experimentation is good, guided experimentation is even better. Especially when it's overseen by an experienced coach.

What To Expect With Intermittent Fasting

Hunger Goes Down

We normally feel hunger pangs about four hours after a meal. So if we fast for 24 hours, does it mean that our hunger sensations will be six times more severe? Of course not.

Many people are concerned fasting will result in extreme hunger and overeating. Studies showed on the day after a one-day fast, there is, indeed, a 20% increase in caloric intake. However, with repeated fasting, hunger and appetite surprisingly decrease.

Hunger comes in waves. If we do nothing, the hunger dissipates after a while. Drinking tea (all kinds) or coffee (with or without caffeine) is often enough to fight it off. However, it is best to drink it black though a teaspoon or two of cream or half-and-half will not trigger much insulin response. Do not use any types of sugar or artificial sweeteners. If necessary, bone broth can also be taken during fasting.

Blood sugar does not crash

Sometimes people worry blood sugar will fall very low during fasting and they will become shaky and sweaty. This does not actually happen as blood sugar is tightly monitored by the body and there are multiple mechanisms to keep it in the proper range. During fasting, the body begins to break down glycogen in the liver to release glucose. This happens every night during our sleep.

If we fast for longer than 24-36 hours, glycogen stores become depleted and the liver will manufacture new glucose using glycerol which is a by-product of the breakdown of fat (a process called gluconeogenesis). Apart from using glucose, our brain cells can also use ketones for energy. Ketones are produced when fat is metabolized and they can supply up to 75% of the brain's energy requirements (the other 25% comes from glucose).

The only exception is for those who are taking diabetic medications and insulin. You MUST first consult your doctor as the dosages will probably need to be reduced while you are fasting. Otherwise, if you overmedicate and hypoglycemia develops, which can be dangerous, you must have some sugar to reverse it. This will break the fast and make it counterproductive.

The dawn phenomenon

After a period of fasting, especially in the morning, some people experience high blood glucose. This dawn phenomenon is a result of the circadian rhythm whereby just before awakening, the body secretes higher levels of several hormones to prepare for the upcoming day -

- Adrenaline - to give the body some energy
- Growth hormone - to help repair and make new protein
- Glucagon - to move glucose from storage in the liver to the blood for use as energy
- Cortisol, the stress hormone - to activate the body

These hormones peak in the morning hours, then fall to lower levels during the day. In non-diabetics, the magnitude of the blood sugar rise is small and most people will not even notice it. However, for the majority of the diabetics, there can be a noticeable spike in blood glucose as the liver dumps sugar into the blood.

This will happen in extended fasts too. When there is no food, insulin levels stay low while the liver releases some of its stored sugar and fat. This is natural and not a bad thing at all. The magnitude of the spike will decrease as the liver becomes less bloated with sugar and fat.

The Best And Worst Types Of Intermittent Fasting, According To Experts

Intermittent fasting requires a lot of discipline and there are some things you should know before giving the buzzy diet a try.

Intermittent fasting may seem like the latest buzzworthy health fad that allegedly aids with weight loss, but experts say it's not all hype. In fact, many experts say the diet can be helpful in boosting longevity, maintaining blood sugar levels, and reaching a healthy weight.

The 1:1 method is the least sustainable fasting method.

Some people overeat on non-fasting days while doing the 1:1 method.

"The least successful variation of fasting is known as the 1:1 method or alternate day fasting."

This type of intermittent fasting entails eating normally for one 24-hour period and then fasting for the next. You should be doing this once or twice a week.

Although this method is becoming popular to kick-start weight loss, it is the least sustainable of all fasting methods in the long-term and has been associated with more overeating on non-fasting days.

The 5:2 fasting method is suitable for those looking for an easier approach to fasting.

A person might feel tired while doing the 5:2 method.

"The 5:2 fasting method requires a person to fast for two non-consecutive days per week". On fasting days, a person consumes no more than 500 to 600 calories. A person might choose this type of fast because it is easier in the sense that they only have to be restrictive once or twice a week.

A major con to the 5:2 fasting method is that it might be very difficult to maintain over the long-term. "The person may feel fatigued, hungry, or irritable on the days that they are consuming so little food, and that could make the workday unpleasant."

The 16:8 method of fasting is one of the easiest forms of intermittent fasting to maintain.

The 16:8 method is the most popular form of fasting.

"The 16:8 method requires a person to eat for eight hours per day and fast for 16 hours (which includes the time a person sleeps) per day." This can be one of the easiest forms of intermittent fasting to maintain, since a person can eat every day, and several meals and snacks can fit inside the eight-hour window. The person can also adjust the window to meet their lifestyle needs and behaviors.

The warrior diet allows you to consume certain fruits and vegetables during the fasting period.

On the warrior diet, some fruits and vegetables are allowed.

"With the warrior diet, a person may consume fruits, vegetables, and liquids with zero (or nearly zero) calories for 20 hours each day."

Those observing this diet are allowed to eat a large meal in the evening.

Overall, intermittent fasting can be good for your gut.

There are some advantages to intermittent fasting, including possible weight loss.

"Intermittent fasting has been shown to increase bacterial diversity and favorably influence the balance of beneficial gut bacteria has been shown to be protective against obesity and weight gain."

Some think, however, that intermittent fasting has mixed findings.

Some think that intermittent fasting isn't any better than traditionally restricting calories.

"Recent studies have found that intermittent fasting has mixed findings and doesn't appear to offer superior metabolic or short term weight control advantages to traditional calorie restriction."

Intermittent fasting can be difficult to maintain long-term.

If you're a snacker, intermittent fasting might not be for you.

No matter what method you choose, intermittent fasting can be difficult to sustain long-term, especially for someone who enjoys eating every few hours.

If you do decide to try intermittent fasting, consult with a dietitian first to get personalized guidance.

Fasting isn't always for everyone.

Pregnant women shouldn't try fasting.

"Fasting is not recommended for pregnant women and for those with eating disorders". "People who need to take medication with food may also have to adjust their window of eating to accommodate this need."

Don't be discouraged to switch to a different fasting protocol.

Find a diet that works for you.

"The most important advice is to find the method that works for you and stay on course, but don't be afraid to switch to a different protocol if you find your original choice doesn't fit your lifestyle."

The benefits are worth the effort and with a little trial and error, results are sure to follow.

The Dangers Of Intermittent Fasting

Studies have shown that intermittent fasting if done incorrectly, can cause a person to have a net gain in weight. When you fast for a couple of days, and then binge on beer and pasta, chances are, you'll do more harm than good.

Intermittent fasting may increase insulin levels, put pancreatic cells at risk, cause unnecessary fatigue, and add to your belly fat. A new study suggests intermittent fasting, while often producing positive results, can harm metabolic health and cause Metabolic Syndrome.

When we have poor metabolic health or Metabolic Syndrome, we are at risk for heart disease, diabetes, and stroke. See your doctor to ensure that you have the proper levels of blood sugar, triglycerides, high-density lipoprotein, and blood pressure.

When you conclude your fast, your body might be oversensitive to the foods you eat. Be aware of your allergies and eat only whole, natural, unprocessed foods, at least for several days. Hydration is the key.

In all fasting, be careful about "starvation mode," when your body starts to conserve energy by reducing the number of calories it burns. Starvation mode is something to avoid. It can cause your body to stop losing weight, and it will most often make you feel depressed, angry, lost, confused or worse. It might also have other negative effects.

Tips For Starting Intermittent Fasting

1. Arm Yourself With Knowledge

Know that you will NOT die if you don't eat for a few hours. If you think what you're doing is harmful or antagonistic to your body, fasting will become a huge hurdle in your mind. Read articles and do research to understand what's actually happening in your body during a fast.

2. Feast Before

Don't commence your fast in a hungry state. If you're going to do the common evening hours or dinner protocol, consider eating A LOT the night before starting. Channel the "I'm so stuffed I could never eat again!" feeling. That way, you won't even be hungry for a substantial part of the first fasting day. Once you've got a day under your belt, you'll be more motivated for day 2, and the days to follow. I find that if I can do something for a day, I can do it many days. It's just making it through the beginning.

3. Fill Your Schedule

Keep your schedule busy during the fasting window. If you've constantly got something to do, you won't be as likely to encounter the all-too-common boredom munchies. Also doing things you love tends to kill appetite anyways. There's a scientific reason for that of course which ties into all of this — I shall post in the future!

4. Stay Active

Keep on moving! Physical activity up-regulates lipolysis and fat burning. It pairs well with fasting, while actually enhancing it! If you simply lie around in a lethargic "I'm fasting" mindset, it'll actually make things more difficult rather than help matters. "Exercise gives you endorphins. Endorphins make you happy. Happy people just don't shoot their husbands, they just don't."

5. Caffeine

In the beginning, caffeine is your friend. Caffeine blunts appetite and increases lipolysis. Drink tea and coffee during the fast — just don't load them with cream and sugar.

6. Remember Sleep Counts

Sleep is not only your health friend in general, it also totally counts towards your fasting window. It's hard to be hungry when you're asleep! Consider timing your sleep to give you a sort of "head-start." For example, if you've settled on an evening feeding window, you could have a big, early dinner the night before fasting. By the time you wake up the next morning, you'll be significantly into your fast already! Also, don't start a fast when you know you'll be sleep deprived, which will only make it unnecessarily difficult.

7. Consider Starting Slow

You can always try just skipping breakfast here and there for starters, and then gradually increase consistency or the fasting window time. "Life moves pretty fast. If you don't slow down and look around, you might miss it."

8. Try Just 3 Days

Committing to an IF pattern for just 3 days will probably get you hooked. If you can make it to day 3, chances are you'll be in LOVE with intermittent fasting by that point and want to go longer. When I started, I said I'd try it for a week (i.e.: weekdays i.e.: 5 days). That was over 3 years ago, and I haven't stopped! (No movie quotes here, just saying that Three Days is officially the biggest tearjerker TV Christmas movie ever).

9. Consider Going Low Carb or Paleo First

Adopting a low carb diet is another way to make your body super fat-efficient. If you're already low carb and "fat adapted," fasting will likely be a breeze from the get-go.

10. See IF as a Learning Experiment, Rather Than a "Test"

When you first start intermittent fasting, don't look at it as a test where you pass or fail. Look at is as a way to experience something new. To see how a different meal pattern feels. To try something different. Rather than thinking "I will do this for a week, otherwise it was pointless," think "I will do this for a week, and then I will know how it feels, and if it is right for me." Experience the moment.

"I don't know if I will have the time to write any more letters because I might be too busy trying to participate….right now these moments are not stories. This is happening….This one moment when you know you're not a sad story. You are alive, and you stand up and see the lights on the buildings and everything that makes you wonder. And you're listening to that song and that drive with the people you love most in this world. And in this moment I swear, we are infinite."

Intermittent Fasting For Women

Intermittent fasting (IF) is the practice of going for prolonged periods without eating.

There are lots of ways to do it, including meal skipping, alternate-day fasting, Eat Stop Eat, and others (PN's free e-book on intermittent fasting offers an excellent rundown).

There's evidence that IF, when done properly, might help regulate blood glucose, control blood lipids, reduce the risk of coronary disease, manage body weight, help us gain (or maintain) lean mass, reduce the risk of cancer, and more.

An accompanying trend that's emerged: While some women who try IF say it's the best thing that's happened to them since grapefruit, others report serious problems, including binge eating, metabolic disruption, lost menstrual periods, and early-onset menopause. This has happened in women as young as their mid-20s.

Maybe my mom was on to something. Maybe IF is totally different for women than for men.

Fasting and female hormones

In the grand scheme of your life's health decisions, experimenting with IF seems tiny, right? Unfortunately — for some women, at least — it seems like small decisions can have big impacts.

It turns out the hormones regulating key functions like ovulation are incredibly sensitive to your energy intake.

In both men and women, hypothalamic-pituitary-gonadal (HPG) axis — the cooperative functioning of three endocrine glands — acts a bit like an air traffic controller.

First, the hypothalamus releases gonadotropin releasing hormone (GnRH).

This tells the pituitary to release luteinizing hormone (LH) and follicular stimulating hormone (FSH).

LH and FSH then act on the gonads (a.k.a. testes or ovaries).

In women, this triggers the production of estrogen and progesterone — which we need to release a mature egg (ovulation) and to support a pregnancy.

In men, this triggers the production of testosterone and sperm production.

Because this chain of reactions happens on a very specific, regular cycle in women, GnRH pulses must be very precisely timed, or everything can get out of whack.

GnRH pulses seem to be very sensitive to environmental factors, and can be thrown off by fasting.

Even short-term fasting (say, three days) alters hormonal pulses in some women.

There's even some evidence missing a single regular meal (while of course not constituting an emergency by itself) can start to put us on alert, perking up our antennae so our bodies are ready to quickly respond to the change in energy intake if it continues.

Maybe this is why certain women do just fine with IF while others run into problems.

Why does IF affect women's hormones more than men's?

We're not totally sure.

But it might have something to do with kisspeptin, a protein-like molecule neurons used to communicate with each other (and get important stuff done).

Kisspeptin stimulates GnRH production in both sexes, and we know it's very sensitive to leptin, insulin, and ghrelin — hormones that regulate and react to hunger and satiety.

Interestingly, females mammals have more kisspeptin than males. More kisspeptin neurons may mean greater sensitivity to changes in energy balance.

This may be one reason why fasting more readily causes women's kisspeptin production to dip, tossing their GnRH off kilter.

Based on what we do know about the HPG axis, kisspeptin, the relationship of hormones to appetite, and women's sensitivity to environmental factors, it's plausible fasting could have a similarly dramatic effect in human females.

Fertility, meet metabolism

You might be thinking: So, what's the big deal if kisspeptin drops off and I miss a few periods? I'm not having kids anytime soon, anyway.

Here's the thing.

The female reproductive system and metabolism are deeply intertwined. If you're missing periods, you can bet a bunch of hormones have been disrupted — not just the ones that help you get pregnant.

Take this snapshot.

In general, women tend to eat less protein than men. Fasting women, obviously, will consume even less.

The Fasted State vs. Fed State

When you eat every few hours, you're in a "fed" state, which is when your body is busy digesting, absorbing, and assimilating the nutrients from your meals. Accelerated fat burning isn't the #1 priority here. Most of us remain in the fed state during the day, aside from when we're sleeping.

The reason why intermittent fasting can provide certain benefits for weight loss is because it allows your body to enter the fasted state, which is when your body's fat burning can really accelerate.

Consuming less protein means taking in fewer amino acids.

Amino acids are needed to activate estrogen receptors and synthesize insulin-like growth factor (IGF-1) in the liver. IGF-1 triggers the uterine wall lining to thicken and the progression of the reproductive cycle.

Hence, low protein-diets can reduce fertility. (Not to mention sexy times.)

And importantly, estrogen isn't just for reproduction.

We have estrogen receptors throughout our bodies, including in our brains, GI tract, and bones. Change estrogen balance and you change metabolic function all over: cognition, moods, digestion, recovery, protein turnover, bone formation...

When it comes to appetite and energy balance, estrogen works in a few ways.

First, in the brainstem, estrogens modify the peptides that signal you to feel full (cholecystokinin) or hungry (ghrelin).

In the hypothalamus, estrogens also stimulate neurons that halt production of appetite-regulating peptides.

Do something that causes your estrogen to drop, and you could find yourself feeling a lot hungrier — and eating a lot more — than you would under normal circumstances.

Estrogens are thus key metabolic regulators.

Yes, estrogens, plural. Because the ratios of the estrogenic metabolites (estriol, estradiol, and estrone) change over time. Before menopause, estradiol is the big player. After menopause, it drops, while estrone stays about the same.

The exact roles of each of these estrogens remain unclear. But some theorize that a drop in estradiol may trigger an increase in fat storage. Why? Because fat is used to make estradiol.

This may partly explain why some women find it harder to lose fat after menopause. And it might serve as a reason to care about your reproductive health — even if you're not focused on making babies.

Men get to walk around looking ripped, and you're struggling to get abs. Well, maybe, evolutionarily speaking, you shouldn't try so hard to get that washboard stomach if you're female.

Low-energy diets can reduce fertility in women. Being too lean is a reproductive disadvantage. Female bodies are exquisitely tuned to any threats to energy and fertility.

When you think about it, this makes good evolutionary sense.

Human females are totally unique in the mammalian world. Get this: Nearly all other mammals can terminate or pause a pregnancy pretty much whenever they need to. You've known this since middle school health class: Female humans can't.

In humans, the placenta breaches the maternal blood vessels, and the fetus is in complete control.

The baby can block the action of insulin in order to hoard more glucose for itself. The fetus can even make the mother's blood vessels dilate, adjusting the blood pressure to get a hold of more nutrients.

That baby is determined to survive no matter what the cost to the mother. This phenomenon, which scientists actually compare to the host-virus relationship, is what's known as "maternal-fetal conflict."

Once a woman becomes pregnant, she can't sweet-talk the fetus to stop growing. The result: Fertility at the wrong time — like, during a famine — could be fatal.

No wonder the reproductive pathway is sensitive to metabolic cues at multiple levels.

How does the body "know"?

OK, so women's hormonal balance is particularly sensitive to how much, how often, and what we eat.

But how do our bodies "know" when food is scarce?

For many years, scientists believed it was a woman's body fat percentage that regulated her reproductive system.

The idea was that if your fat reserve dipped below a certain percentage (somewhere around 11 percent might be a reasonable guess), hormones would get messed up and your period would stop. Boom: no risk of pregnancy.

This makes a lot of sense. If there isn't much to eat, you'll lose body fat over time.

But the situation is actually more complicated than that. After all, food availability can change quickly. And — as you probably know if you've ever tried to lose weight — body fat often takes a while to drop, even if you're eating fewer calories.

Meanwhile, women who aren't especially lean can also stop ovulating and lose their periods.

That's why scientists have come to suspect overall energy balance may be more important to this process than body fat percentage per se.

Stressors and energy balance

Specifically, negative energy balance in women may be to blame for the hormonal domino effect we've been talking about. And it's not just about how much food you eat.

Negative energy balance can result from:

- Too little food
- Poor nutrition
- Too much exercise
- Too much stress
- Illness, infection, chronic inflammation
- Too little rest and recovery

Heck, we can even use up energy reserves by trying to keep warm.

Any combination of these stressors could be enough to put you into negative energy balance and stop ovulation: training for a marathon and nursing a flu; too many days in a row at the gym and not enough fruits and vegetables; intermittent fasting and busting your butt to pay the mortgage.

You're thinking, did she just reference paying the mortgage?

You bet. Psychological stress can absolutely play a role in damaging our hormonal equilibrium.

Our bodies can't tell the difference between a real threat and something imaginary generated by our thoughts and feelings. (Such as worrying about how you're going to get abs.)

The stress hormone cortisol inhibits our friend GnRH, and suppresses the ovaries' production of estrogen and progesterone.

Meanwhile, progesterone is converted to cortisol during stress, so more cortisol means less progesterone. This leads to estrogen dominance in the HPG axis. More problems.

You could be hovering at 30 percent fat. But if your energy balance is negative for a long enough time, especially if you're stressed, reproduction stops.

That's the theory, anyway.

What to do now

Based on what we know, intermittent fasting probably affects reproductive health if the body sees it as a significant stressor.

Anything that affects your reproductive health affects your overall health and fitness.

Even if you don't plan to have kids.

But intermittent fasting protocols vary, with some being much more extreme than others. And factors such as your age, your nutritional status, the length of time you fast, and the other stresses in your life—including exercise—are also likely relevant.

So. Is fasting for you?

Considering how much remains unclear, I would suggest a conservative approach.

If you want to try IF, begin with a gentle protocol, and pay attention to how things are going.

Stop intermittent fasting if:

- Your menstrual cycle stops or becomes irregular
- You have problems falling asleep or staying asleep
- Your hair falls out
- You start to develop dry skin or acne
- You're noticing you don't recover from workouts as easily
- Your injuries are slow to heal, or you get every bug going around
- Your tolerance to stress decreases
- Your moods start swinging
- Your heart starts going pitter-patter in a weird way
- Your interest in romance fizzles (and your lady parts stop appreciating it when it happens)
- Your digestion slows down noticeably
- You always seem to feel cold
- Fasting is not for everyone

The truth is, some women should not even bother experimenting. Don't try IF if:

- You're pregnant
- You have a history of disordered eating
- You are chronically stressed
- You don't sleep well
- You're new to diet and exercise

Pregnant women have extra energy needs. So if you're starting a family, fasting is not a good idea.

Pros and Cons of Intermittent Fasting for Women

Some of the benefits of intermittent fasting may include:

- Sustainable weight loss
- An increase in lean muscle mass
- More energy
- An increase in cell stress response
- A reduction in oxidative stress and inflammation
- Improvement around insulin sensitivity in overweight women
- Increased production of neurotrophic growth factor (which could boost cognitive function)

Now, here's the tricky part. Although intermittent fasting may have its benefits, women are naturally sensitive to signs of starvation, so intermittent fasting for women is a whole different beast.

When the female body senses it's headed towards famine, it will increase the production of the hunger hormones, ghrelin and leptin, which signal the body that you're hungry and need to eat. Additionally, if there's not enough food for you to survive, your body is going to shut down the system that would allow you to create another human. This is the body's natural way of protecting a potential pregnancy, even if you're not actually pregnant or trying to conceive.

It's not that you're intentionally imposing a famine upon yourself — but your body doesn't know that. It doesn't know the difference between true starvation and intermittent fasting, which is why it defaults to this protective mechanism.

Therefore, some of the cons due to hormonal imbalances brought on by intermittent fasting may also lead to:

- Irregular periods (or complete loss of period)
- Metabolic stress
- Shrinking of the ovaries
- Anxiety

- Fertility issues
- Difficulty sleeping

Since all of your hormones are so deeply interconnected, when one hormone is thrown off balance, the rest are also negatively impacted. It's like a domino effect. As the "messengers" that regulate nearly every function in your body — from energy production to digestion, metabolism, and blood pressure — you don't want to disrupt their natural rhythm.

With all of these drawbacks, you may be wondering: could you (and would you still want to) practice intermittent fasting as a female? If you take a more relaxed approach, the answer is yes. When done within a briefer timeframe, intermittent fasting may still help you reach your weight loss goals and provide the other benefits previously mentioned, without messing up your hormones.

The Best Intermittent Fasting Methods for Women

Clock

So, what exactly is a relaxed approach to intermittent fasting? Again, since there's little research done on intermittent fasting, we're dealing with a bit of a gray area. The opinions also tend to vary depending on which site you visit, or which health expert you ask. From what we've found, the general guidelines to brief intermittent fasting for women are:

- Do not fast for longer than 24 hours at a time
- Ideally fast for 12 to 16 hours
- Do not fast on consecutive days during your first two to three weeks of fasting (for instance, if you do a 16-hour fast, do it three days a week instead of seven) Drink plenty of fluids (bone broth, herbal tea, water) during your fast
- Only do light exercise on fasting days, such as yoga, walking, jogging, and gentle stretching

Options for Intermittent Fasting

There are several different intermittent fasting methods discussed online. Here are a few of the most popular ones.

Crescendo Method

The Crescendo Method is one of the best ways to ease into intermittent fasting without shocking your body or aggravating your hormones. It doesn't require you to fast every day, only a few days per week, spaced throughout the week. For example, Monday, Wednesday and Friday.

Fasting Window: 12-16 hours

Eating Window: 8-12 hours

Safe for Women: Yes

16/8 Method

The 16/8 method, sometimes called the "leangains method," is another brief intermittent fasting routine that's used specifically to target body fat and improve lean muscle mass (a.k.a. your gains!).

Fasting Window: 16 hours

Eating Window: 8 hours

Safe for Women: Yes

24 Hour Protocol (a.k.a. "Eat-Stop-Eat")

The 24 hour protocol, also known as "eat-stop-eat" requires you to do a 24-hour fast, once or twice a week. You can choose the time you start fasting. Some people prefer to fast from 8 pm to 8 pm the following day, or begin their fast after breakfast.

Fasting Window: 24 hours

Eating Window: 0

Safe for Women: Yes, when done a maximum of 2 times per week.

The 5:2 Diet

The 5:2 diet, also known as the "Fast Diet," involves restricting calories two days a week to 500 calories per day (with two 250 calorie meals), while eating normally for the other five days. For example, you might eat all of your regular meals Saturday through Wednesday, and eat 500 calories per day on Thursdays and Fridays. There isn't a ton of research to back up this diet, although it was publicized by Michael Mosley, a British journalist and doctor. Since it doesn't completely restrict food on the fasting days, it may also be an effective way to ease into fasting without shocking your system. The Fast Diet is considered safe for men and women.

Fasting Window: No fasting window, just calorie restriction to 500 calories per day for 2 fasting days per week

Eating Window: Assume regular caloric intake 5 days per week

Safe for Women: Generally considered safe for women, but studies are lacking on this diet

Additionally, intermittent fasting is meant to complement a healthy diet and lifestyle — not act as a way to remedy five days of eating nutritionally-bankrupt foods, such as refined sugar, processed foods and fast foods.

Intermittent fasting may work amazingly well for some people, and terribly for others. Most importantly, if you do decide to give intermittent fasting a try, be sure to listen to your body's feedback. Easing into intermittent fasting by starting with shorter fasting windows can help with initial symptoms of hunger and discomfort. But if it becomes too uncomfortable, be honest with yourself, accept it, and move on.

How Women Can Use Intermittent Fasting Safely

This doesn't mean women have to miss out on the benefits of intermittent fasting. Instead, I recommend that women follow some simple rules when it comes to intermittent fasting. This will help you tap into the many benefits associated with intermittent fasting while sidestepping the risks.

- Don't fast on consecutive days
- Instead, pick no more than two or three non-consecutive days in a week to practice intermittent fasting
- Don't fast for more than 12 or 13 hours at a time. Going any longer can trigger a negative hormonal cascade
- Don't do intense workouts on fasting days
- Don't fast when you're bleeding

- During your eating window, choose the best diet for your hormonal health

If you give this slow and steady approach to intermittent fasting a try for a couple months and feel great, you can consider going for a longer window of time each day without eating (up to 16 hours), but pay close attention to how you feel and drop back to a smaller window—or stop intermittent fasting all together—if you start experiencing symptoms of hormone imbalance

If you start to experience symptoms of hormone imbalance while intermittent fasting, or if the hormone imbalance symptoms you already experience get worse, stop fasting right away. These symptoms include:

- Your period becomes irregular or stops
- You start having problems sleeping or falling asleep
- You notice changes in metabolism and digestion
- You feel moody or experience brain fog
- You notice negative changes in how your hair and skin looks
- You're always cold

Intermittent Fasting For Women Over 50

For women who are interested in weight loss, intermittent fasting may seem like a great choice, but many people want to know, should women fast? Is intermittent fasting effective for women? There have been a few key studies about intermittent fasting which can help to shed some light on this interesting new dietary trend.

Obviously our bodies and our metabolism changes when we hit menopause. One of the biggest changes that women over 50 experience is that they have a slower metabolism and they start to put on weight. Fasting may be a good way to reverse and prevent this weight gain though. Studies have shown that this fasting pattern helps to regulate appetite and people who follow it regularly do not experience the same cravings that others do. If you're over 50 and trying to adjust to your slower metabolism, intermittent fasting can help you to avoid eating too much on a daily basis.

When you reach 50, your body also starts to develop some chronic diseases like high cholesterol and high blood pressure. Intermittent fasting has been shown to decrease both cholesterol and blood pressure, even without a great deal of weight loss. If you've started to notice your numbers rising at the doctor's office each year, you may be able to bring them back down with fasting, even without losing much weight.

Intermittent fasting may not be a great idea for every woman. Anyone with a specific health condition or who tends to be hypoglycemic should consult with a doctor. However, this new dietary trend has specific benefits for women who naturally store more fat in their bodies and may have trouble getting rid of these fat stores.

Weight Loss Tips For Women

Diet and exercise may be key components of weight loss for women, but many other factors play a role.

In fact, studies show that everything from sleep quality to stress levels can have a major impact on hunger, metabolism, body weight, and belly fat.

1. Cut Down on Refined Carbs

Refined carbs undergo extensive processing, reducing the amount of fiber and micronutrients in the final product.

These foods spike blood sugar levels, increase hunger, and are associated with increased body weight and belly fat.

Therefore, it's best to limit refined carbs like white bread, pasta, and prepackaged foods. Opt for whole-grain products like oats, brown rice, quinoa, buckwheat, and barley instead.

2. Add Resistance Training to Your Routine

Resistance training builds muscle and increases endurance.

It's especially beneficial for women over 50, as it increases the number of calories that your body burns at rest. It also helps preserve bone mineral density to protect against osteoporosis.

Lifting weights, using gym equipment, or performing body-weight exercises are a few simple ways to get started.

3. Drink More Water

Drinking more water is an easy and effective way to promote weight loss with minimal effort.

According to one small study, drinking 16.9 ounces (500 ml) of water temporarily increased the number of calories burned by 30% after 30–40 minutes.

Studies also show that drinking water before a meal can increase weight loss and reduce the number of calories consumed by around 13%.

4. Eat More Protein

Protein foods like meat, poultry, seafood, eggs, dairy, and legumes are an important part of a healthy diet, especially when it comes to weight loss.

In fact, studies note that following a high-protein diet can cut cravings, increase feelings of fullness, and boost metabolism.

One small 12-week study also found that increasing protein intake by just 15% decreased daily calorie intake by an average of 441 calories — resulting in 11 pounds (5 kg) of weight loss.

5. Set a Regular Sleep Schedule

Studies suggest that getting enough sleep may be just as crucial to losing weight as diet and exercise.

Multiple studies have associated sleep deprivation with increased body weight and higher levels of ghrelin, the hormone responsible for stimulating hunger.

Furthermore, one study in women showed that getting at least seven hours of sleep each night and improving overall sleep quality increased the likelihood of weight loss success by 33%.

6. Do More Cardio

Aerobic exercise, also known as cardio, increases your heart rate to burn extra calories.

Studies show that adding more cardio to your routine can result in significant weight loss — especially when paired with a healthy diet.

For best results, aim for at least 20–40 minutes of cardio per day, or around 150–300 minutes per week.

7. Keep a Food Journal

Using a food journal to track what you eat is an easy way to hold yourself accountable, and make healthier choices.

It also makes it easier to count calories, which can be an effective strategy for weight management.

What's more, a food journal can help you stick to your goals, and may result in greater long-term weight loss.

8. Fill up on Fiber

Adding more fiber to your diet is a common weight loss strategy to help slow the emptying of your stomach and keep you feeling fuller for longer.

Without making any other changes to diet or lifestyle, increasing dietary fiber intake by 14 grams per day has been associated with a

10% decrease in calorie intake and 4.2 pounds (1.9 kg) of weight loss over 3.8 months.

Fruits, vegetables, legumes, nuts, seeds, and whole grains are all great sources of fiber that can be enjoyed as part of a balanced diet.

9. Practice Mindful Eating

Mindful eating involves minimizing external distractions during your meal. Try eating slowly and focusing your attention on how your food tastes, looks, smells, and feels.

This practice helps promote healthier eating habits and is a powerful tool for increasing weight loss.

Studies show eating slowly can enhance feelings of fullness and may lead to significant reductions in daily calorie intake.

10. Snack Smarter

Selecting healthy, low-calorie snacks is a great way to lose weight and stay on track by minimizing hunger levels between meals.

Choose snacks high in protein and fiber to promote fullness and curb cravings.

Whole fruit paired with nut butter, veggies with hummus, or Greek yogurt with nuts are examples of nutritious snacks supporting long-lasting weight loss.

11. Ditch the Diet

Although fad diets often promise quick weight loss, they can do more harm than good when it comes to your waistline and your health.

For example, one study in college women showed eliminating certain foods from their diet increased cravings and overeating.

Fad diets can also promote unhealthy eating habits and lead to yo-yo dieting, both of which are detrimental to long-term weight loss.

12. Squeeze in More Steps

When you're pressed for time and unable to fit in a full workout, squeezing more steps into your day is an easy way to burn extra calories and increase weight loss.

In fact, it's estimated non-exercise-related activity may account for 50% of the calories your body burns throughout the day.

Taking the stairs instead of the elevator, parking further from the door, or taking a walk during your lunch break are a few simple strategies to bump up your total number of steps and burn more calories.

13. Set Attainable Goals

Setting SMART goals can make it easier to reach your weight loss goals while also setting you up for success.

SMART goals should be specific, measurable, achievable, relevant, and time-bound. They should hold you accountable and lay out a plan for how to reach your goals.

For example, instead of simply setting a goal to lose 10 pounds, set a goal to lose 10 pounds in 3 months by keeping a food journal, going to the gym 3 times per week, and adding a serving of vegetables to each meal.

14. Keep Stress Under Control

Some studies suggest increased stress levels can contribute to a higher risk of weight gain over time.

Stress may also alter eating patterns and contribute to issues like overeating and binging.

Exercising, listening to music, practicing yoga, journaling, and talking to friends or family are several easy and effective ways to lower stress levels.

15. Try HIIT

High-intensity interval training, also known as HIIT, pairs intense bursts of movement with brief recovery periods to help keep your heart rate elevated.

Swapping cardio for HIIT a few times per week can amp up weight loss.

HIIT can decrease belly fat, increase weight loss, and has been shown to burn more calories than other activities, such as biking, running, and resistance training.

16. Use Smaller Plates

Switching to a smaller plate size may help promote portion control, aiding weight loss.

Although research remains limited and inconsistent, one study showed that participants who used a smaller plate ate less and felt more satisfied than those who used a normal-sized plate.

Using a smaller plate can also limit your portion size, which can reduce your risk of overeating and keep calorie consumption in check.

17. Take a Probiotic Supplement

Probiotics are a type of beneficial bacteria that can be consumed through food or supplements to help support gut health.

Studies show probiotics can promote weight loss by increasing the excretion of fat and altering hormone levels to reduce appetite.

In particular, Lactobacillus gasseri is a strain of probiotic that's especially effective. Studies show it can help decrease belly fat and overall body weight.

18. Practice Yoga

Studies show that practicing yoga can help prevent weight gain and increase fat burning.

Yoga can also decrease stress levels and anxiety — both of which may be tied to emotional eating.

Additionally, practicing yoga has been shown to reduce binge eating and prevent preoccupation with food to support healthy eating behaviors.

19. Chew Slower

Making a conscious effort to chew slowly and thoroughly can help increase weight loss by cutting down on the amount of food you eat.

According to one study, chewing 50 times per bite significantly decreased calorie intake compared to chewing 15 times per bite.

Another study showed that chewing food either 150% or 200% more than normal reduced food intake by 9.5% and 14.8%, respectively.

20. Eat a Healthy Breakfast

Enjoying a nutritious breakfast first thing in the morning can help start your day off on the right foot and keep you feeling full until your next meal.

In fact, studies find that sticking to a regular eating pattern may be linked to a reduced risk of binge eating.

Eating a high-protein breakfast has been shown to decrease levels of the hunger-promoting hormone ghrelin. This can help keep appetite and hunger under control.

21. Experiment With Intermittent Fasting

Intermittent fasting involves alternating between eating and fasting for a specific window of time each day. Periods of fasting typically last 14–24 hours.

Intermittent fasting is thought to be as effective as cutting calories when it comes to weight loss.

It may also help enhance metabolism by increasing the number of calories burned at rest.

22. Limit Processed Foods

Processed foods are typically high in calories, sugar, and sodium — yet low in important nutrients like protein, fiber, and micronutrients.

Studies show consuming more processed foods is associated with excess body weight — especially among women.

Therefore, it's best to limit your intake of processed foods and opt for whole foods, such as fruits, vegetables, healthy fats, lean proteins, whole grains, and legumes.

23. Cut Back on Added Sugar

Added sugar is a major contributor to weight gain and serious health issues, such as diabetes and heart disease.

Foods high in added sugar are loaded with extra calories but lacking in the vitamins, minerals, fiber, and protein your body needs to thrive.

For this reason, it's best to minimize your intake of sugary foods like soda, candy, fruit juice, sports drinks, and sweets to help promote weight loss and optimize overall health.

Intermittent Fasting Meal Recipes

Stuffed Mushrooms

Three medium Portobello mushrooms - 250g = 55 calories

Low-fat ricotta cheese - 100g = 116 calories

Low fat grated cheddar cheese - 40g = 130 calories

Boneless leg ham 30g = 45 calories

Chopped parsley - 1/4 cup = 5 calories

Diced red capsicum - 20g = 8 calories

Preparation:

Pre-heat oven to 180 degrees Celsius

Remove the stems from the mushrooms and dice them

Finely cut the ham

Combine the ham, capsicum, parsley, ricotta cheese and diced mushroom stems in a bowl and mix well

Spoon the above mixture into the inverted mushrooms

Sprinkle with the grated cheese

Cook in pre-heated oven still at 180 degrees Celsius for 20 minutes

Mushroom Delight

Mushrooms are very low in calories, but very filling.

260g chopped Portobello mushrooms

75g chopped green beans

50g grated zucchini

1 spring onion

2 large eggs (90g each)

5g minced garlic

10g wholegrain mustard

10g grated cheese

Mix all ingredients except cheese and eggs in a non-stick frying pan and cook for 5 to 10 minutes on high heat (no oil is needed as the mushrooms will lose water, which will flow into the frying pan).

Add eggs and cook for a further 1-2 minutes

Remove from heat and serve with cheese sprinkled on top

Total calories: approximately 270.

Slendier Noodles Carbonara

Slendier noodles are very filling and nutritious but best of all they contain only 8 calories per 100 grams!!

250g packet of Slendier noodles (20 calories)

150mls low-fat thickened cream,

bacon with the fat removed,

parmesan cheese to taste,

rice bran cooking spray to cook the bacon.

Instructions:

Cut the bacon into small pieces and fry it in cooking spray or a very small amount of cooking oil

Add thickened cream and leave to boil for a couple of minutes to make sauce

Remove sauce from heat

Prepare noodles as per instructions on packet

Add sauce to noodles and mix together

Add parmesan cheese to taste, but be sure to measure how much you're adding so you can work out how many calories are in it.

Cook noodles as per instructions on packet

Weigh your ingredients first to work out the amount of calories in this delicious dish. For me, it added up to 320 calories.

Clear Mushroom Soup

Ingredients:

Thick cut Portabello, Field and Shitake mushrooms (enough to satisfy).

Two cloves garlic.

Five cut shallots.

Two small chillis.

Two spring onions, thin sliced.

Method:

Lightly fry in deep pot with a tiny spray of oil.

Add 500 ml of either Chicken, Beef or Vegetable stock.

Ground pepper to taste.

Bring to boil, then simmer 20 mins or as desired.

This meal is usually around 100 calories depending on quantities.

How To Do Intermittent Fasting For Weight Loss

Intermittent fasting is a powerful tool for successful and sustained weight loss.

Fasting gets you into ketosis quicker — it drains your glucose reserves, forcing your body to reach into its fat stores for energy.

If you really want to lose fat, intermittent fasting is the perfect tool. Research shows that intermittent fasting — cycling in and out periods of fasting and eating — has huge benefits for your body and brain. It can ward off chronic disease, improve memory and brain function, and boost your energy levels. What's more, intermittent fasting is a powerful hack for losing weight quickly, and keeping it off.

Intermittent fasting can fast-track your weight loss goals by busting stubborn fat, reducing calories, and rewiring your metabolism for better performance. Read on for the science behind intermittent fasting and weight loss, how to maximize your fast, and a sample schedule to start you off.

When you're intermittent fasting, you eat all the food your body needs but during a shorter period of time. There are many methods, but the most common involves eating during a 6- to 8-hour window, and fasting the remaining 14 to 16 hours.

Intermittent fasting also succeeds where many weight-loss regimes fail: by targeting and reducing visceral fat. Visceral fat is the stubborn, internal fat packed deep around your abdominal organs. During a period of six months, people on an intermittent fasting diet were able to shed four to seven percent of their visceral fat.

How does intermittent fasting boost weight loss?

If you think about it, fasting isn't all that unnatural. Your ancestors evolved to thrive in situations when food was scarce. On top of a slew of other health benefits, intermittent fasting triggers a perfect storm of metabolic changes to tackle weight loss and fat reduction. How does it work?

The fat-busting benefits of intermittent fasting include:

Kickstarts ketosis: Usually, reaching full ketosis takes careful planning and extreme carb limiting, but intermittent fasting provides a shortcut to this fat-burning state. Once your body drains glucose — its primary source of energy — it is forced to burn through its fat reserves for energy in a process called ketosis. Ketosis improves your blood chemistry, reduces inflammation, and helps you drop weight fast. To really burn through extra fat, combine your intermittent fasting with a keto diet. Learn more here about why keto is more effective with intermittent fasting

Lowers insulin levels: Intermittent fasting acts on insulin in two ways. First, it boosts your adiponectin levels, which helps restore insulin sensitivity to prevent weight gain and diabetes. Second, fasting decreases your fasting insulin levels. Lowered insulin is the cue your body needs to make the switch to burning stored fat instead of glucose.

Improves cholesterol: Intermittent fasting diets impact cholesterol by decreasing your levels of LDL and VLDL cholesterols (the bad stuff). While improving your cholesterol won't directly lead to weight loss, overweight and obese people are more likely to have dangerously high LDL and VLDL cholesterol, and the cardiovascular risk that comes with it.

Reduces inflammation: Lowering inflammation is key to losing weight, boosting longevity, and reducing your risk of major illnesses such as Alzheimer's and cancer. That's why it's at the core of the Bulletproof Diet. Intermittent fasting decreases oxidative stress and inflammation across the board, including inflammatory markers such as adiponectin, leptin, and brain-derived neurotrophic factor.

Boosts metabolism: Intermittent fasting also boosts protein, fat, and glucose metabolism in animal studies. Boosting your resting metabolism helps your body burn more calories throughout the day, even while you rest. Fasting also increases your levels of adrenaline and noradrenaline, hormones that help your body free up more stored energy (that's your body fat) during a fast.

The Best Intermittent Fasting Weight Loss Strategy

The human body was designed very efficiently for times of scarcity and stress. Food scarcity was a common reality and the body has developed specific pathways to be very efficient in times of fasting. In times of stress, for survival purposes we adapted a fight or flight mode that forces us to work out bodies at a very high-intensity for a relatively short period of time.

The combination of intermittent fasting and high intensity exercise promotes fat burning hormones that improve tissue healing and metabolic processes. In this chapter you will learn intermittent fasting weight loss strategies using time restricted feeding and high intensity exercise.

Our long-ago ancestors had to struggle daily for adequate food sources. They most often grazed on wild berries, herbs, raw nuts & seeds as they foraged through the woods during the day. At night, they would relax with the latest kill eating most-often a high protein, high fat burning meal. This sort of diet was dependent upon the success of their hunting endeavors.

Fasting was a regular way of life for our ancestors. This is evident with the positive adaptations the body goes through during the fasting periods. Fasting allows our body to go into a catabolic (tissue breakdown) period without promoting inflammatory conditions. This enables the bodily resources to eliminate older, damaged cells and replace them with stronger cellular components

Today, fasting is not a regular way of life, but we can use fasting for a wide variety of health conditions. Fasting weight loss strategies should be implemented with high intensity exercise for the best results.

High Intensity Movement is a Way of Life

High intensity exercise was a necessity of life for our ancestors as they chased down and killed animals for food. Many cultures battled with other cultures regularly. The fight or flight lifestyle was quite evident and it was almost always at 90-100% of maximal intensity.

Anything less than this could quite often lead to death or starvation. This way of life led to a lean and incredibly strong body. Most men had body fat under 10% while women typically ranged between 10-20%. They were also able to produce incredible muscular forces to overcome obstacles with their battle trained bodies.

To have high-quality of life in the 21st century, we must understand and work in harmony with our bodies' primitive past. Intermittent fasting and high-intensity, short durational exercise are genetic requirements that help our bodies thrive, adapt and evolve with better survival characteristics. This includes a strong fit muscular system, a titanium immune system and an efficient digestive tract.

Fasting & Fitness Boost HGH:

Intermittent fasting for periods ranging from 12-24 hours along with high intensity exercise has a positive effect on boosting human growth hormone (HGH). HGH is a very important protein based hormone that is produced by the pituitary gland. HGH enhances the cellular repair processes that allow us to age with grace. HGH regulates metabolism for fat burning, muscle building, and slow-down the negative effects of stress.

Researchers at the Intermountain Medical Center Heart Institute found that men who had fasted for 24 hours had a 2,000% increase in circulating HGH. Women who were tested had a 1,300% increase in HGH.

A study showed that lactic acid accumulation helps to trigger HGH. Lactic acid is only produced in response to intense anaerobic training. Aerobic training is not intense enough to produce the kind of lactate triggering of HGH.

Long-Duration Training Can Be Damaging:

Low-intensity, long duration aerobic training is catabolic in nature. This means it produces lots of free radicals without promoting significant amounts of repair peptides, enzymes and fat burning hormones.

The net effect is a wearing down of bodily resources. High-intensity training also produces free radicals but it triggers an abundance of repair peptides, enzymes and hormones to be released. The net effect of this is healthy tissue repair and favorable effects on body composition and anti-aging qualities.

The Best Fasting Weight Loss Strategy

For the best results with intermittent fasting weight loss techniques it is recommended that exercising 4 days per week after having water or fat fasted for 12-16 hours. This means you miss either dinner the night before and drink a lot of water and coffee (and you can do grass-fed butter and MCT oil in your coffee if you like) and exercise about an hour after rising in the morning.

Otherwise, you consume dinner the night before but fast through breakfast (other than lots of water and possibly a fat fuel coffee or keto matcha green tea) and then you exercise around lunch time. Hydrate after your exercise session and then having a protein shake about 30-60 mins after you finish your exercise.

For many, as they get more accustomed to the intermittent fasting are able to wait a few hours after their workout before they eat. I typically like to tell people to wait until you are hungry after your exercise session to consume food as this is a more advanced way to boost human growth hormone production.

Over time, you may notice you are able to go 18-20 hours without consuming carbohydrate or protein and exercise right at the end of your fast. This peak fasting exercise session can have a profound impact on your growth hormone production and be an amazing stimulus for fasting weight loss.

The key is to stay hydrated and use some pink salts to keep your mineral balance in order. You can also do some diluted broth and some fat burning coffee or keto matcha green tea to keep your energy up while fasting.

The Stages Of Intermittent Fasting

Intermittent fasting works for men and women. Here's how to make it work for you too...

You've heard all about intermittent fasting.

You know the benefits.

You've read the success stories.

But you're not quite sure how to get started. Or, you've started but now your progress has stalled.

Stage 1: Skip Breakfast

This is the jumping off point for most people new to the practice of intermittent fasting.

By simply skipping breakfast, you extend the amount of time in the fasted state from roughly 8 hours to 12 hours.

The hardest part about this change is mental – most of us have heard for years that "breakfast is the most important meal of the day" or that skipping breakfast is a big dietary no-no because it will crash your metabolism (myths, by the way.)

Once you've mastered this stage, you will realize the conventional wisdom regarding the importance of breakfast is dead wrong (as conventional wisdom often is). With nothing more than a cup of coffee to start your day, you will enjoy increased fat burning and more free time in the mornings.

Side note: 90% of people who start intermittent fasting begin by skipping breakfast. This works fine for most people. But in some rare cases, an individual may be better served by eating breakfast and instead skipping lunch. This includes individuals who engage in strenuous early morning training sessions or those who simply find lunch inconvenient.

Overall, this is a relatively simple dietary adjustment for most people. The first few days may be difficult but most people will adapt within a week. After that first week, your desire for breakfast will typically be gone and you will be surprised at how much time, energy and financial resources you've invested in breakfast over the years.

Stage 2: Extend the Fast to 16 Hours

After a couple weeks in Stage 1, most people are ready for Stage 2. In this stage, we extend the fast from roughly 12 hours to approximately 16 hours.

Based on the popular lean gains template, this results in 16 hours of daily fasting and an 8 hour daily eating window. Typically this means skipping both breakfast and lunch and breaking the fast with an early dinner around 4 pm.

So fasting from midnight to 4pm (16 hours) and then breaking the fast at that point. Obviously the schedule will shift based on what time you STOP eating at night. But the breakdown should remain the same: 16 hours of fasting and an 8 hour eating window.

This is a big increase in time spent in the fasted state. For the first time in most people's lives, they will actually spend more hours per day NOT eating than eating. (A 2:1 ratio of fasting versus fed.)

For this reason, the degree of difficulty jumps during this stage. But as the difficulty increases, so does the fat loss. For many people, this is all they need to get their ideal physique. They fast for 16 hours, eat anything they want for 8 hours and they stay lean without counting calories, carbs or stressing about following a formal "diet."

Expect to remain at this stage for at least a month. Most people are able to see slow and steady fat loss for multiple months at this stage.

Side note: Stage two is where most people get stuck.

When fat loss stalls, it's time for…

Stage 3: Eat Once Per Day

When stage #2 no longer serves your purpose, the next step is to again extend the fasting period from 16 hours a day to roughly 20 hours a day.

For most people this essentially works out to eating one main meal per day (typically at night), although the "meal" will commonly be drawn out into a 4-hour eating window.

Based on the Warrior Diet template, the results from this stage can be dramatic. At this stage, most people are able to obtain the necessary leanness to finally see abs (sub 10% body fat for men, sub 18% body fat for women.)

Another benefit to this stage is that you do not need to eat perfectly "clean" to enjoy rapid weight loss. In fact some people may NEED to incorporate junk food (or at least healthy, higher calorie foods like nuts and oils) in order to maintain their weight at this stage.

Expect to stay at this stage for at least 1-2 months. Expect to fall off the wagon from time to time as this schedule can be difficult to maintain.

Stage 4: Eat Once Per Day, Whole Foods Only

The beauty of stage 3 is that you can lose weight even while eating less-than-perfectly. Pizza, chicken nuggets, fries, milk shakes – when you're eating only once per day you can get away with a lot and still lose weight.

However, if weight loss stalls in stage 3 than it's time to make the next logical jump: Eat once per day and start to clean up your diet. This means making a concentrated effort to eat only whole foods – eggs, beef, chicken, veggies, fruits, grains, cheese, etc.

It doesn't take a rocket scientist to figure out if something qualifies as a "whole food." Just cut out the processed junk, cut out the sugars and sweets, and weight loss will pick up again.

Again, you don't have to over-think this. There is no need to over-analyze things to death and drive yourself batty wondering if walnuts qualify as a whole food or if oatmeal is good or bad.

If it walks on the farm or grows in the ground, you're good to go.

If it's widely considered "junk food" (pizza, ice cream, chips, pop, etc) than it's off limits.

Of course this does not mean you can't ever have pizza again. It just means most of the time your daily meal should be based around whole foods. If you need a rule of thumb, shoot for 6 days of clean eating with only one "junk food" meal per week.

99% of people will never need to go beyond Stage #4. When combined with a proper resistance training program, stage #4 can get you to 8% body fat (for men) or 15% body fat for women which gives you the lean physique most people are striving for.

Stage 5: Incorporate Weekly 44 Hour Fasts

Stage 5 is an advanced strategy reserved for those seeking rare levels of leanness (sub 7% body fat for men, sub 12% body fat for women), or those with a deadline driven fat loss goal.

After your last meal on Sunday night, you do not eat again until Tuesday evening. This results in a 40-48 hour fast at the beginning of the week. If you eat only one meal per day – consisting of whole foods – during the rest of the week, you should achieve your physique goals within a short time.

Most people will not need to use this strategy every single week. Often times it will be used for a few consecutive weeks leading up to a vacation or photo shoot. Or it will be used 1-2 times a month for maintenance.

Side Effects Of Intermittent Fasting

You've heard so much about the benefits of intermittent fasting (IF), including weight loss, reduced inflammation, improved digestion, reduced bloating, increased mental clarity, better sleep, and getting a handle on sugar cravings.

You're ready to give it a try, but you need to be aware of some not-so-awesome side effects that you'll likely experience in the beginning. "Think about it this way - people don't go from couch potato to triathlete overnight. Your body needs time to acclimate to any extreme changes. So you're going to experience some side effects when you suddenly stop eating for long periods of time." These can be unbearable at the beginning, but as long as you know how to deal with them, you'll be able to stick with IF and reap all the benefits.

Before starting any new diet plan, including intermittent fasting, be sure to check in with your doctor first.

Hunger

When you're used to eating five to six times a day, your body comes to expect food at certain times. "The hormone ghrelin is responsible for making us feel hungry. It typically peaks at breakfast, lunch, and dinner time and is partially regulated by food intake. When you first start fasting, ghrelin levels will continue to peak and you will feel hungry." At first, it will take serious willpower. Days three through five may feel the worst, but there will come a time when you reach the beginning of your eating window and you don't even feel hungry!

Combat hunger in that first week or two by drinking tons of water to keep your belly full, help you feel more alert, and help satiate that habit of having to put something in your mouth. Within 30 minutes of waking up, pound at least 12 ounces. If you feel a pang of hunger, drink another 12 ounces or more. One thing intermittent fasting will teach you is that what you thought was hunger was probably thirst or boredom.

Drinking black coffee and tea can also curb hunger. Also get enough sleep, keep busy, and avoid strenuous workouts in the first couple weeks, since that can increase hunger. Eating enough the day before and getting your fill of carbs, healthy fats, and protein is also key in preventing hunger.

Cravings

"If I told you that you couldn't eat watermelon ever again, chances are, all you'd want to do is eat a slice of watermelon. During intermittent fasting, you're going extra long periods without eating. So chances are, you'll only be able to think about eating. That's when the cravings kick in. You'll also find that you're more likely to crave sweets and/or refined carbohydrates because your body is looking for that glucose hit."

Do whatever you can to not think about food, and be sure to indulge a little during your feeding window so you have the chance to satisfy those cravings.

Headaches

As your body is getting used to this new eating schedule, dull headaches that come and go are pretty common. Dehydration can be one factor, so make sure you're drinking tons of water during both your fasting and feeding windows.

Headaches can also be caused by blood sugar levels decreasing and by stress hormones released by your brain while fasting. With time, your body will get used to this new eating schedule, but try to remain as stress-free as possible.

Low Energy

Your body is no longer getting the constant source of fuel you used to get from eating all day long, so expect to feel a little sluggish those first couple of weeks. Try to keep your day as relaxed as possible so you can exert the least amount of energy. You might want to give your workouts a break or just do light exercise like walking or yoga. Getting extra sleep may also help.

Irritability

Feeling hangry is real, and it sucks. Expect to feel a little cranky when your blood sugar levels drop or you're dealing with the other side effects of IF, like cravings and low energy. You can deal with this by avoiding situations and people that might make you more annoyed and focusing on doing things that make you happy.

Heartburn, Bloating, and Constipation

Your stomach produces acid to help digest your food, so when you're not eating, you may experience heartburn (this side effect isn't as common as the others). This could range from mild discomfort to burping all day to full-on pain. Time should cure this side effect, so just keep drinking water, prop yourself up when you sleep, and when you do eat, avoid greasy, spicy foods that could make your heartburn worse. If it doesn't go away, speak to your doctor.

Intermittent fasting can also cause constipation, which can cause bloat and discomfort.

Feeling Cold

Cold fingers and toes while fasting is pretty common, but for a good reason! When you fast, blood flow increases to your fat stores. Called adipose tissue blood flow, this helps to move fat to your muscles, where it can be burned as a fuel. When your blood sugar decreases, that can also make you more sensitive to feeling cold. Combat coldness by sipping hot tea, taking warm showers, wearing extra layers, and avoiding being outside in the cold for prolonged periods of time.

Overeating

People tend to overeat in the beginning of the IF journey, either because they heard calories don't matter (they do!) or because they are so excited about food that they overdo it. Planning out your meals ahead of time can keep portions in check.

You may also feel so famished by the time your fasting window ends that you eat really fast and end up eating way more than you normally would. "When the fasting period is over during IF, you need to be mindful about your first meal. You may feel like reaching for a slice a pizza (or four), but opt for the grilled chicken and salad instead. Your future self will thank you."

Bathroom Trips

Because you're drinking oceans of water to stay hydrated and fill you up, you're going to feel the need to run to the bathroom more often. We're talking maybe even twice an hour! Sorry to say there's no way around this. You definitely don't want to reduce your water intake, so just make sure you're always close to a bathroom.

All of this sounds pretty bad, but these symptoms generally only last a week, maybe three at most. The best way to alleviate the side effects is to ease into intermittent fasting - don't go from eating six meals a day to eating two. "Just give it some time and intermittent fasting becomes natural and healthy, with less appetite, more mental sharpness, and an enviable waistline in the long run."

Always Listen to Your Body

"Intermittent fasting is not for everyone. For example, people with diabetes, pregnant or nursing mothers, and children should not practice intermittent fasting. People who are managing chronic illnesses should always check in with their doctor prior to starting any new diet or eating regime. Finally, anyone with a history of or risk for developing eating disorders should avoid fasting of any kind."

There is a time when these side effects shouldn't be ignored. "IF might not be for you if you experience dizziness due to low blood sugar, if fasting is interfering with your ability to keep up with your responsibilities, or you develop an unhealthy obsession with food." You may need to cut your fast short and eat earlier than you planned, or you may need to stop fasting altogether. If you have any concerns or issues, it's always a good idea to consult your doctor.

Conclusion

In the most simple sense, intermittent fasting is rotating between periods of eating, and periods of not eating. I'll list the benefits below, but the general reasoning behind participating in Intermittent fasting (IF) is that many people respond very well to eating most of their calories in less meals, especially while dieting.

This allows for hunger control, insulin sensitivity (read: muscle building) and more time for burning fat (increased adrenaline/noradrenaline).

You might fast through your sleep and into the afternoon, and then have a window of eating that lasts a few hours. In this period you would also have the workout.

Or it could mean that you wake up and eat a large meal, and fast late into the day until second/last meal.

Be smart and efficient, choose a program that gets you results with researched efficient methods. Either way the responsibility is taken at your leisure, but to squeeze the most results out of any method you choose, do your research and listen to your body.